THE PROSTATE BOOK

The
PROSTATE
BOOK

Sound Advice on Symptoms and Treatment

Newly Revised and Updated

STEPHEN N. ROUS, M.D.

Illustrations by Betty Goodwin

W·W·NORTON & COMPANY

New York   London

The text of this book is composed in Baskerville,
with display type set in Friz Quadrata.
Composition by Sue Carlson
Manufacturing by The Maple-Vail Book Manufacturing Group.

Library of Congress Cataloging-in-Publication Data
Rous, Stephen N. (Stephen Norman), 1931–
The prostate book : sound advice on symptoms and treatment /
Stephen N. Rous. ; illustrations by Betty Goodwin.
          p.   cm.
"Newly revised and updated."
Includes index.
ISBN 0-393-05010-6
1. Prostate—Popular works. I. Title.
RC899 .R672 2001
616.6'5—dc21   00-052714

W. W. Norton & Company, Inc.
500 Fifth Avenue, New York, N.Y. 10110
www.wwnorton.com

W. W. Norton & Company Ltd.
Castle House, 75/76 Wells Street, London W1T 3QT

1 2 3 4 5 6 7 8 9 0

This book,
with all of my love,
is for
Margot, Ben, David, and Elizabeth.

Contents

Acknowledgments

Writing a book like this is undeniably a good deal of work, but it is a labor well repaid because it will hopefully help men who are suffering from one or another disease of the prostate to better understand the problem and their choices of treatment for this problem. Moreover, writing a book such as this has been enjoyable because of the help and the cooperation of colleagues with whom I have worked at one stage or another of my career. In that vein I would like to express my deep appreciation to several of these colleagues who have been of immeasurable help to me as I wrote various portions of this book.

Dr. Michael Blute, professor and chair of urology at the Mayo Clinic, and Dr. Horst Zincke, professor of urology at the Mayo Clinic, were most helpful in providing various bits of information regarding radical prostatectomy and hormone therapy in the treatment of prostate cancer. Dr. Reza Malek of the Mayo Clinic and Dr. Barry Stein, chair of urology at Brown University, were both generous in sharing their knowledge about laser treatment of the prostate gland. Dr. Robert Amdur, professor of radiology at the University of Florida, is a colleague with whom I worked most intimately when he was at Dartmouth, and I thank him for helping me with his fount of knowledge about radiation therapy for prostate cancer; also Dr. E. Ann Gormley, another Dartmouth colleague, was most gracious in explaining the ins and outs of urodynamics testing. I would like to thank Dr. Judd Moul of the Walter Reed Army Medical Center, who kindly shared his extensive knowledge about PSA determinations and PSA testing with me, and also Dr. Nancy Dawson, formerly of the Walter Reed Army Medical Center and now a professor of medicine at the University of Maryland, who was kind enough to bring me up to date on the newest happenings in the treatment of advanced prostate cancer. From my former institution, the Medical University of South Carolina, I want to thank the late Dr. Robert Nelson, professor of urology, as well as Dr. Pamela Ellsworth, assistant professor of urology and my Dartmouth colleague, for their help in bringing me up to date regarding the newest treatments for erectile dysfunction. Also from the Medical University of South Carolina, I am indebted to Dr. Nancy Curry, professor of radiology, for allowing me to use most, if not all, of the x-rays and CT scans included in this book. Ms. Betty Goodwin, former chief of medical illustrations at the Medical University of South Carolina, was able to turn my not very well expressed thoughts and ideas into beautiful drawings that perfectly illustrate what I had hoped to illustrate.

Finally, I am truly and totally indebted to Susan Pullen, my secretary at the Medical University of South Carolina who is now retired and living happily in the mountains of North Carolina. Mrs. Pullen was responsible for transcribing every word in this book, all the earlier editions of this book, and virtually every other book I have ever written, and she never lost her cool as she revised manuscripts countless times. Her many excellent suggestions were gratefully accepted, and I will always appreciate her incredible efficiency and her superb cheerfulness as she labored at her word processor for many, many hours. She is truly a unique individual, and in the many years before and since I met this wonderful woman, I have never been fortunate enough to work with anyone even half as capable, as competent, and as delightful!

Introduction

I am often asked by lay people to describe my specialty of urology. The best answer that I have been able to come up with is that urology is the medical and surgical treatment of diseases of the urinary tract in men, women, and children and of the reproductive tract in males. I then sometimes add that these many and varied diseases occur in all age groups, from the newborn to the very aged. Before I can say very much more about my favorite subject, I am usually interrupted by a man saying, "Urology? The urinary tract? The reproductive tract? That must mean that you know all about the prostate, too. Listen, I hate to talk shop outside of office hours, but could you just explain why it is that . . . "

The man with the problem is not very different from most men that I have met in forty years of practicing urology. Without a doubt, the prostate gland seems to generate more questions, more misunderstandings, more concern, and more anxieties than any other part of the male genitourinary tract. This really isn't at all surprising, though, because the prostate gland does indeed cause more grief for more men than just about any other structure in the body, and the symptoms and difficulties arising from the prostate cover almost the entire adult life of a man.

When I was originally asked by my publisher back in 1987 if I would be willing to write a book about the prostate, I quite literally jumped at the opportunity to do so, because I have found that a major part of practicing the specialty which I love so much is taken up by patients with prostate problems. At least daily, I find myself explaining to patients why their prostate gland is causing them grief, discussing the rationale for my recommended treatment, whether medical or surgical, and particularly dispelling the many myths and outright false-hoods that patients have learned about the prostate gland. I was therefore happy to write such a book for the benefit of my patients and the patients of my colleagues. Perhaps this book should even have been dedicated to all those men who have ever suffered from any prostatic diseases and perhaps to those men who will yet suffer the misery of their afflictions.

If you are reading this book, I imagine that you have been told that you have a disease of your prostate gland, or perhaps you think that you may have such a disease, or perhaps you know someone afflicted with one of the maladies of the prostate. In this book I will try to help you understand your prostate as fully as possible so you and your doctor will hope-fully be able to overcome your problem, handle your problem, or at the very least learn to live with your problem.

There are three distinct and different types of diseases that affect the prostate gland, and they occur, for the most part, at different periods of a man's life. Infection and inflam-mation of the prostate tend to occur at a relatively young age, and most men with this problem are between the ages of 25 and 45. The second of the diseases affecting the prostate is benign prostatic hyperplasia, usually known simply as BPH, which generally begins to produce symptoms at about age 45 or 50. The disease BPH is extremely common, and it is prob-able that most men in the United States who are over the age of 50 have at least some of the symptoms of this condition. The last of the conditions affecting the prostate is cancer, which is uncommon before age 50 but which then increases in fre-quency as a man gets older. Prostate cancer is the most com-mon cancer in U.S. men (excluding skin cancer) and the second (to lung cancer) most common cause of cancer deaths. In this book I will discuss each of these three distinct condi-tions at length so you will understand fully the symptoms that they produce, the various tests that I feel should be used in their diagnosis, and the specific forms of therapy that I have found to be most effective in each of these groups of condi-tions.

I have learned that the prostate gland in many ways is dif-ferent from other structures of the body that are prone to the same types of diseases. Most men think of the prostate gland as a genital, or sexual, structure, and I suppose that this is so in the strictest sense of the words since the main function of the prostate is to produce the fluid in which spermatozoa travel to the outside of the body during orgasm and ejaculation. Unfortunately, however, because of this perception of the prostate as a sexual structure, I have found that most men tend to be extraordinarily frightened about prostatic disease of any kind. They are generally much more worried than I might otherwise expect them to be only on the basis of their symptoms. I am constantly amazed at the widespread prevalence of the firm belief that prostatic infection or inflammation, or even BPH, will lead to that most feared of all conditions, the inability to achieve an erection! This one single fear I have found to be an overriding concern to virtually all men. I have found this fear to be partly based on the dismal prospect of not being able to have sexual intercourse, but I have also found that to most men the potential to perform sexual intercourse is just as important as the act itself because these men feel that they cannot possibly be true men if they cannot perform sexually.

If there is anything that I have learned from patients in forty years, it is that treating their physical ailments is simply not sufficient when these ailments are prostatic in origin. Whatever extra time is required to put the disease in perspective, to explain exactly what the disease is, and particularly to reiterate time and again that these prostatic problems are not related to the ability to perform sexually, has all been time extremely well spent. It has been estimated that about half of all complaints bringing patients to primary care physicians are psychosomatic in origin. While I do not believe this figure to be nearly that high with urological problems presented to a urologist, I am totally and absolutely convinced of the necessity of recognizing the mental anguish and outright fear of many of my patients and of taking whatever time is necessary to address these concerns, to allay these fears, and to reassure my patients that their dreaded presentiments will not materialize.

Because diseases of the prostate gland are so very widespread and prevalent, I have found that most of them are initially treated by a primary care physician. This is often perfectly satisfactory initially and in cases where a patient responds rapidly to therapy. However, for those patients with infection or inflammation that does not improve, for those patients with the symptoms of BPH, and particularly for those patients with prostatic cancer, I feel that the best form of therapy is that given by a urologist.

Since that statement is a very strong one, I should tell you why I have said it. Only a urologist has had the extensive and excellent training required to care for these complex urologic diseases. The training of the urologist is a long and arduous one, extending for five and very often six years following graduation from medical school. This training is carried out in one of approximately 120 approved programs in the United States, and it invariably is in a highly specialized university medical center. During the course of these five or six years, the embryo urologist, who is known as the urology resident, is exposed to the entire spectrum of urologic diseases. He or she is taught urologic diagnosis and treatment by professors of urology in these university medical centers, many of whom are truly distinguished educators and clinicians. The educational process of the urology resident is a step-by-step one culminating in the final year of training in which the resident is actually responsible for the medical and surgical treatment of large numbers of patients, always under the supervision of a university faculty member.

At the completion of the last year of residency training, known as the chief resident year, the embryo urologist (who is now 31 or 32 years of age) sits for a two-day written Part I examination that is given by the American Board of Urology and covers all the aspects of urology that have been studied during the previous five or six years, including interpreting the various imaging studies and diagnosing various GU conditions from a photograph of the microscopic appearance of various surgical specimens. After completing the residency, the new urologist is now permitted to practice urology in a community of her or his choosing where she or he is constantly monitored by other urologic colleagues in the community and by the senior urologist at the hospital in which patient care is delivered.

Assuming that the new urologist practices competent urology as determined by a group of peers in the same community, and assuming that the Part I examination was passed, he or she is then allowed to take the oral examinations of the American Board of Urology which are given approximately eighteen months after the written examination. The oral examinations are administered by at least two very senior academic urologists who are invariably professors of urology at their own universities. These oral examinations, which can cover several hours, probe deeply into the abilities of the newly minted urologist to solve various clinical problems that are presented by the examiner. Satisfactory completion of Part II of the examination entitles the new urologist to be a diplomate of the American Board of Urology. Receipt of this prestigious and coveted certificate means that the individual physician can then truly be considered an expert and a specialist in urologic diseases. There are fewer than 10,000 practicing physicians in the United States who have earned this privilege.

Urology, like virtually all other branches of medicine, is an art as well as a science. This means, among other things, that the treatment of patients is not necessarily a set thing where *A* will always follow *B* as it would in a pure science. There are often many treatment options for the same disease because no one treatment exists that works 100 percent of the time. Similarly, even the diagnostic steps taken in determining why a patient has such and such symptoms are not always cut and dried and are not always the same steps that would be taken in the same situation by every other physician.

Different physicians who are equally bright and equally capable will follow different diagnostic routes to the same end and will use different methods of treating the same disease. No physician is necessarily wrong, for the differences reflect the fact that in the hands of a given physician one treatment has consistently shown better results than another, and physicians will have differing experiences that will lead to different conclusions. Throughout this book, I have frequently expressed my own opinions about the diagnosis and treatment of many urologic problems. However, my opinions are just that and certainly are not meant in any way to imply that others who may differ with me are wrong.

Finally, I hope that this book will fulfill the expectations of my readers; I will be satisfied if it serves to comfort and to reassure those men suffering from the various diseases of the prostate.

THE PROSTATE BOOK

1

Normal Anatomy and Normal Function

I have always found the study of anatomy to be tedious. It involves rote memory work without the necessity of thinking very much. I have also come to realize that an intimate knowledge of anatomy is not at all necessary for internists or family physicians, but it really is very important for surgeons who must make daily use of this knowledge.

I also believe that some very basic knowledge of anatomy and the normal function of the prostate will help you to better understand any difficulty that you may be having and the treatment of that difficulty.

The normal prostate gland in the adult male lies between the urinary bladder and the external urethral sphincter, the muscle that a man tightens when he wants to shut off his flow of urine (Fig. 1–1). The adult prostate gland is about the size and shape of a large chestnut and it weighs about 20 grams, or a little less than 1 ounce. At the time of birth, the prostate is about the size of a pea. It gradually increases in size until puberty; then there is a period of rapid growth that continues until the third decade of life when the prostate reaches its normal adult size. The size of the prostate gland then remains constant until about age 40 or 45, at which time benign

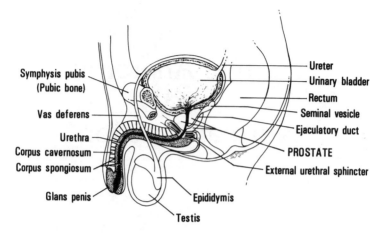

Figure 1–1   *The entire male genitourinary tract. This figure shows the relationship of the prostate gland to the urinary bladder and the external urethral sphincter. It also illustrates the other genitourinary tract structures. This is a lateral view taken through the precise midpoint of the male body.*

prostate hyperplasia (BPH) commences in most men. BPH is the process of aging in the presence of the male hormone (testosterone) in which the prostate gland enlarges by a multiplication of its cells and which is usually, but not always, accompanied by symptoms of difficulty voiding. This growth will continue very slowly until death. In a relatively few, very fortunate men, BPH just does not develop; these men will never have any of the symptoms commonly associated with this condition. In these very few and lucky men, the prostate slowly decreases in size over the remaining years of life, a condition that is normal for these men.

The anatomic fact that I have found most confusing to patients and even to some physicians may also be confusing to you. I refer to the relationship of the prostate gland to the prostatic urethra, of the prostatic urethra to the rest of the urethra, and of the prostate gland to the bladder. The way that I have found best to simplify this is to ask you to think of the prostate gland as an apple with the core removed (Fig. 1–2). The prostatic urethra is then that portion of the urethra which

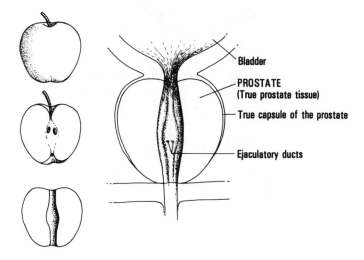

Figure 1–2   *The prostate gland. This shows the prostate looking like an apple which has been cut in half with the core removed.*

is within the prostate gland and has precisely the same anatomic relationship to the gland as the core of the apple has to the apple itself. The entire urethra is a channel through which urine flows when it leaves the bladder; the prostatic urethra is the first part of that channel (Fig. 1–3). The prostatic urethra ends at the external urethral sphincter. This is the sphincter muscle which you voluntarily contract when you want to suddenly stop your flow of urine while voiding. The very small portion of the urethra that passes through the external sphincter muscle is known as the membranous urethra. The next part of the urethra going from the bladder to the penis is known as the bulbous urethra. The last and often the longest portion of the urethra is external and is known as the penile or the pendulous urethra. You will note that the internal portion of the urethra may at times be almost as long as the external portion. To say it once again, the prostatic urethra is nothing more than a straight channel through the prostate gland by way of which urine flows as soon as it leaves the bladder.

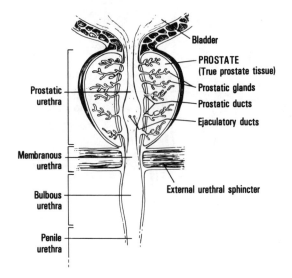

Figure 1–3   *The relationship of the prostate gland to the prostatic urethra and to each of the other portions of the urethra.*

If you were to look at your prostate under a microscope, you would see that it is composed of muscle, glands, and fibrous or connective tissue. The same types of tissue make up benign prostatic hyperplasia when it arises. The only difference between the normal prostate tissue and the BPH tissue is that the latter generally has more muscle and fibrous tissue in proportion to glandular tissue than the normal prostate does.

There are many, many small glands within the prostate, and each of these pours its secretion into one of the prostatic ducts during orgasm and ejaculation. These ducts in turn empty into the prostatic urethra. The ducts that carry the spermatozoa also empty into the prostatic urethra; these are called the ejaculatory ducts. These ducts, in addition to bringing the spermatozoa into the prostatic urethra, also bring fluid from the seminal vesicles which are saclike structures, two in number, directly behind the base of the bladder. The seminal vesicles serve as a storage area for spermatozoa and provide some of the fluid that serves as a nutrient for the spermatozoa. The vast majority of the sperm reach the ejaculatory ducts via the vas deferens which are paired, cordlike structures, through which the sperm are transported from the testis and epididymis. It is these vas deferens structures that are surgically divided during the very popular contraceptive operation known as a vasectomy. During orgasm, spermatozoa, fluid from the seminal vesicles, and fluid from the prostate gland all pour into the prostatic urethra because of contractions of the muscles of the prostate and the seminal vesicles. This mixture of fluids is then propelled to the outside during ejaculation because of the spasmodic contractions of the muscles that surround the urethra.

The prostate is referred to as an accessory sex gland. It is considered to be an accessory (and not a primary) part of the sexual or reproductive tract because, even though its sole function is sexual, it is only indirectly involved in procreation. Obviously, the testes are the site of the manufacture of spermatozoa and the penis is necessary to deliver the spermatozoa into the upper reaches of the vagina. The testes and the penis are therefore considered to be the primary sexual structures. The prostate is considered to be a gland because it produces secretions and thereby meets the definition of a gland. These secretions are manufactured within the prostate gland and enter the prostatic urethra along with fluid from the ejaculatory ducts, at the time of orgasm and ejaculation (Fig. 1–4). All of these secretions then go to the outside of the body during ejaculation, and so the prostate is known as an externally secreting gland. In contrast, the male body has endocrine glands such as the testis, the adrenal, and the pituitary, all of which produce internal secretions that go throughout the body via the bloodstream.

The principal function of the prostate is to produce the fluid that makes up much of the semen. The primary purpose of this fluid is to serve as a vehicle in which the spermatozoa can travel to the outside at the time of ejaculation. Prostatic fluid secondarily provides some nourishment to the spermatozoa.

An understanding of the male reproductive system will be helpful to you so that you can better place the role of the prostate in its proper perspective (Fig. 1–5). Each testis is located in the scrotum and has two principal functions, both of which are controlled by hormones from the pituitary gland. First, the testis manufactures the spermatozoa needed for pro-

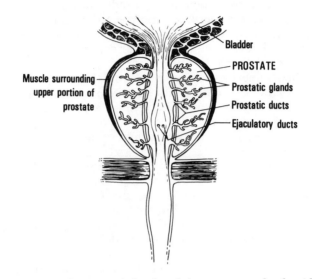

Figure 1–4   *The prostate gland and the numerous glands within the prostate with the relationships of these glands to the prostatic ducts shown. Note the presence of the ejaculatory ducts, which empty into the prostatic urethra from the vas deferens and the seminal vesicles.*

creation. This is done in very small tubules within the testis known as seminiferous tubules. The testis also manufactures almost all of the body's principal male hormone, testosterone. This is produced by the Leydig cells which are also within the testis. These cells discharge the testosterone directly into the bloodstream. For this reason, the testis is considered to be an endocrine gland. The spermatozoa which are manufactured in the testis converge into a network of ducts which then lead into the epididymis, a structure which is just behind the testis and connected to it by means of a network of ducts (the rete testis).

The epididymis is a long, coiled tubular structure which provides a storage place for the spermatozoa to mature and then go on their way when needed. The vas deferens are a pair of small and heavily muscled tubular structures that convey spermatozoa from the epididymis to the seminal vesicles and ejaculatory ducts. These in turn empty into the prostatic

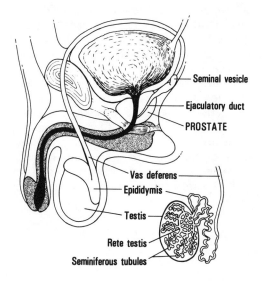

Figure 1–5 *The male reproductive system, with details of the testis and the relationships of the testis to the epididymis, to the vas deferens, to the seminal vesicle, and to the ejaculatory duct shown.*

urethra at the time of orgasm and ejaculation. The muscles of the vas deferens serve to propel the spermatozoa in their journey toward the prostatic urethra. The seminal vesicle itself is a paired structure that is really little more than a storage sac located behind the base of the bladder. It manufactures and stores a nutrient fluid for the spermatozoa to use during their journey through the urethra, into a woman's vagina, uterus, and up into the fallopian tubes in order to fertilize an ovum. Spermatozoa are also stored within the seminal vesicles. How much gets stored is a function of the frequency of ejaculation.

During sexual stimulation, the penis becomes erect because of an increased flow of blood into the paired, spongy bodies (corpora cavernosa) that lie within the penis. At the height of sexual excitement, orgasm takes place, a phenomenon produced by muscular contractions that propel spermatozoa and fluid from the prostate and seminal vesicles into the prostatic urethra and then to the outside of the body, known as ejaculation. The strong muscles that surround the prostate and urethra propel the ejaculate to the outside, while at the same time the bladder neck closes to prevent the ejaculated fluid from going back into the bladder. Of the total amount of fluid in the ejaculate, something under 5 percent contains spermatozoa; the remainder is made up of fluid from the prostate gland and from the seminal vesicles. A very small component of the ejaculate is fluid from the small glands that surround the urethra. The prostate makes and stores its secretions more or less continuously, and for all practical purposes, these secretions are never totally emptied from the prostate. The production of fluid will vary with demand, which in turn is a function of the frequency of ejaculation and therefore the status of the fluid within the prostate at any given time.

2

How the Doctor Diagnoses Your Problems

From the earliest days of medical school we doctors have been told to "listen to the patient if you want to know what is wrong with him." I agree with this completely, and I have found that I can usually form an accurate impression of my patient's problem simply by listening to him relating his symptoms and by then knowing which questions to ask in order to home in on a tentative diagnosis. This process is known as "taking a history" from a patient.

I next examine my patient placing particular emphasis on those details of the physical examination which I think will yield the most information, on the basis of the historical information I have already received. As it usually turns out, the combination of a well-taken history and a good physical examination of the genitourinary tract are sufficient for me to reach a provisional diagnosis of the cause of my patient's problem. For most patients, though, what I *think* is the cause of their problem is not sufficient; they want me to be absolutely certain of the diagnosis that I give to them.

Diagnosing with precision the various disorders of the prostate can be a tricky business, but we urologists happily have at our disposal a large variety of diagnostic tests that we can administer. From these many tests, though, only a few are chosen, and I will always try to choose the *fewest* possible studies needed in order to be absolutely certain of my diagnosis. I look on these diagnostic studies that I do obtain as very necessary in order to confirm the provisional diagnosis that I have made from the history and physical exam. Occasionally, though, the diagnostic studies serve to refute my provisional diagnosis and force me to rethink it.

I fully recognize that you, as the patient, may have considerable dismay about the various tests that we urologists do. This is not only because of the natural aversion that many people have to physicians and their tests but because of the very intimate area of the body with which we urologists deal. I assure you that we do the absolute minimum number of studies compatible with reaching a correct diagnosis, and I further assure you that virtually all the studies done by urologists are far more unpleasant to contemplate than they are to undergo! Discussed below are several of the most frequently done diagnostic studies, but always remember that you will most likely only need to have a very few of these.

Examination of the Urine

This single test probably provides more information about a patient and his genitourinary tract per dollar of cost than any other. It is really a screening test since it alone does not provide any definitive diagnoses but rather serves as a red flag alerting a physician to look further. Although urinalysis is able to detect sugar in the urine of diabetic patients, the parts of the urinalysis that are directly related to prostatic diseases are the microscopic examination and the culture of the urine. The microscopic part of the urine examination is helpful in a patient with prostatic disease since it will show white blood cells (pus cells) which may be indicative of infection. It can also demonstrate the presence of red blood cells which may be due to an insignificant problem such as a mild inflammation in the urethra or bladder or may be an early sign of a life-threatening tumor. Anything over 0-3 red blood cells per high-power microscopic field is generally considered to be abnormal, although certainly not necessarily serious.

The culture of the urine is absolutely necessary if infection in the urinary tract is to be diagnosed with any certainty. Any microscopic exam of the urine showing more than three white blood cells per high-power field is generally considered to be abnormal, although not necessary indicative of any disease. Just as often as not, these few white blood cells in the urine represent contamination, for example, as from the penis in an uncircumcised man. The presence of these white blood cells, however, should suggest at least the possibility of infection in the urinary tract although I feel it is incorrect to make a definite diagnosis of infection without culturing the urine.

A urine culture should ideally be obtained from the middle portion of the urinary stream, after a man retracts his foreskin and cleans the glans penis well with soap and water. A circumcised man does not usually need to do this cleaning procedure. Midstream urine is obtained by having a man start to void the first few ounces of urine into the toilet, then collect the middle portion of his stream into a sterile container, and then finish emptying his bladder directly into the toilet. *At no point from beginning to end of this process should the urinary stream be stopped or interrupted.* One milliliter of the urine obtained from the middle portion of the urinary stream is then transferred to a small dish which contains a nutrient on which bacteria (if present) will grow when placed in an incubator at a temperature that is suitable for bacterial growth. After twenty-four hours of incubation, any bacteria present in the urine can be identified by its growth pattern in the dish, and the number of bacteria present per milliliter of urine can be counted. At the same time as the cultures are being done, small cardboardlike discs, impregnated with various antibiotics, are placed in a section of the dish to see which antibiotics are effective against any bacteria that may be growing. It usually takes about a day for a urine culture and bacterial sensitivity study to be done. This study should always be done before a diagnosis of an infection is made, even though an infection may be suspected and treatment started on the basis of the patient's symptoms and the presence of white blood cells in the urine.

Blood Tests to See How Well the Kidneys Are Working

Two of the blood tests that are commonly used to measure kidney function are known as urea nitrogen and creatinine. When the kidneys are functioning normally, these tests have normal values, but when there is diminished kidney function, the blood levels of urea nitrogen and creatinine will often rise to abnormal levels. Urea is formed normally in the liver from the breakdown of protein, and it is then found in the blood as urea nitrogen, or blood urea nitrogen (BUN) as it is more commonly known. Normally, most of the urea nitrogen is excreted in the urine; its level in the blood will be abnormally high if the kidneys are not working well enough to excrete it in normal amounts. The urea nitrogen levels can also be raised or lowered by abnormalities within the body that have nothing whatever to do with kidney function. For example, since urea is formed within the liver, it can be depressed to extremely low levels if the patient suffers from liver failure and is therefore not able to manufacture urea. Such might be the case even if the kidney function were also severely diminished, and the result could then be a perfectly normal urea nitrogen level even though kidney function was severely diminished. However, the creatinine level in the blood is generally not dependent on any bodily functions other than the kidney function. For this reason, then, the creatinine level of the blood is a much more accurate measurement of kidney function than is the urea nitrogen level. Creatinine is produced from the normal breakdown of body muscles; this is the reason that a heavily muscled man will have a higher, but perfectly normal, creatinine level than a very small man with minimal muscle mass. All of the creatinine that is made is removed from the blood by kidneys and excreted in the urine.

Abnormal elevations of the creatinine (and the urea nitrogen as well) generally *do* indicate a decrease in kidney function, but this is not necessarily irreversible or permanent. For example, if there is obstruction of urine from both kidneys—as there might well be from a very large prostate gland that is preventing the bladder from emptying—the blood creatinine level might be elevated because the kidneys cannot function normally in the face of the obstruction. Once the blockage of the kidneys is relieved, the blood creatinine level may well return to normal. Whether it does is determined by how normal the kidneys were before the obstruction occurred and how long the obstruction was present. It should be noted, relative to the blood creatinine level, that if only one-half of one kidney is functioning normally, the blood creatinine level will still be in the normal range. In other words, the human body has a great deal of reserve renal function.

Normal creatinine levels vary with age and muscle mass,

but in the adult male the level is generally between 1.2 and 1.4 milligrams per 100 milliliters of blood. This may be somewhat lower in very small men and it normally rises slightly in men over age 60.

Blood Tests That Suggest the Possibility of Prostate Cancer

Prostate specific antigen, or PSA, is very likely the best tumor marker in all of medicine although it most definitely cannot by itself diagnose prostatic cancer if it has an elevated value or eliminate the possibility of prostate cancer if it has a normal value. This blood test came into common clinical usage in the late 1980s, and it has been used with increasing frequency ever since, perhaps even to the point of inappropriate use.

Prostate specific antigen is a substance that is produced by the glandular cells of normal, enlarged, and malignant prostate tissue. Therefore, it should be obvious that this PSA blood test cannot, by itself, either diagnose or eliminate the possibility of prostate cancer because it is not specific for prostate cancer. Because benign prostatic tissue makes PSA and because the prostate tends to enlarge with advancing age, it is perfectly understandable that PSA levels may increase somewhat with aging. As a result of measuring the PSA blood levels in very large groups of men, with and without known prostate cancer, suggestions as to upper limits of normal for various age groups have been made (Table 2–1).

Table 2–1		
Age	**Whites (ng of PSA/ml)**	**African Americans (ng of PSA/ml)**
40–49	0.0–2.5	0.0–2.0
50–59	0.0–3.5	0.0–4.0
60–69	0.0–3.5	0.0–4.5
70–79	0.0–3.5	0.0–5.5
Age-Specific Reference Ranges for Normal Values of the PSA Test		

Source: Walter Reed Army Medical Center data based on PSA levels in 3,500 men without prostate cancer.

Other evaluations of the PSA levels of large groups of men have suggested that men in their seventies might have somewhat higher upper limits of permissible PSA levels.

The difference between the two numbers in the limits is the difference between sensitivity (the lower limit) and specificity (the upper limit). In other words, using the lower limit would increase the likelihood of detecting prostate cancer at an earlier stage following prostate biopsies, but it would also lead to more negative biopsies which some might consider to be unnecessary biopsies. The higher limit for a PSA would lead to a greater yield of positive prostate biopsies, but these cancers might well be in a more-advanced stage. More and more urologists are leaning toward using the lower limits of acceptability for PSA levels as seen in the table (Table 2–1) and this is particularly true for younger patients. Certainly, patients in their forties with a PSA that is over 2.0–2.5 represent a potentially worrisome situation, and this is so because it is these younger patients in their forties and fifties in whom prostate cancer represents a grave threat to their ability to live out a normal life span. It is these patients in their forties and fifties who are most in need of treatment for their prostate cancers, and therefore I feel it is indeed a wise course to use a very low threshold of PSA level to trigger a prostate biopsy which could in turn diagnose these prostate cancers. Men over 70, on the other hand, do not always need any form of treatment for prostate cancer since their life expectancies are not too different whether or not prostate cancer is present.

My general rule of thumb is that if a man has an estimated ten years or more of life expectancy, I will recommend treatment for prostate cancer if it is present. In practice, then, for most of my patients, this means that if a man is over 70, I will usually not recommend any treatment unless he obviously has the genes for longevity or unless he indicates that he definitely wants to be treated regardless of his age.

I have already indicated that prostate cancer cannot be diagnosed by the PSA level alone, and this is because the level can be raised to what might be considered a worrisome level simply by a very large benign prostate, by infection in the prostate or in the bladder, by infarction of a portion of the prostate, or by as yet unknown but albeit extremely rare other causes. Since there are other factors, as just noted, that can elevate the PSA level, how does the urologist decide when to pursue the matter and recommend a prostate biopsy and when to recommend simply continued observation? You should realize that although benign and malignant prostate tissue both manufacture PSA in the glands of the prostate, malignant cells make up to ten times as much PSA as do benign cells per gram of prostate tissue, and therefore the higher the PSA level, the greater the likelihood there is of prostate cancer's existing. Since it turns out that most PSA elevations seen in common clinical practice by urologists have PSA levels that are less than 9 or 10, the resulting biopsies of the prostate triggered by these PSA elevations are most often negative for prostate cancer.

Although there is no additional blood test at the present time that can definitively say whether a PSA elevation represents cancer in the prostate, there are some other factors that can be helpful in determining the need for a prostate biopsy. First, and most obvious, is the digital rectal examination (see Chapter 4) because if this is abnormal in any way, so as to suggest the possibility of prostate cancer, a biopsy should be seriously considered regardless of the PSA level.

Also, a number known as the PSA density may be helpful in certain instances although certainly not definitive. The PSA density concept is based on the fact that, per gram of prostate tissue, cancer cells will make more PSA than benign cells will. When an ultrasound examination of the prostate is done (see below), it is possible to determine the size (in cubic centimeters) and the weight (in grams) of the entire prostate. The PSA density is then calculated by dividing the PSA value by the weight of the prostate in grams. If the number resulting from this calculation (the PSA density) is 0.10 or less, the odds are greatly against the presence of cancer. If the PSA density is 0.15 or less, the odds are still somewhat against the presence of prostate cancer. On the other hand, if the resulting PSA density is 0.2 or higher, the odds of cancer's being present in the prostate are significantly increased. The concept of PSA density is an interesting one; it is also logical because it is based on the truism that the higher the PSA value per weight of the prostate gland, the greater the chances of cancer. However, I must again emphasize that neither the PSA nor the PSA density is able, by itself, to say with any degree of certainty that prostate cancer is present. The definitive diagnosis of this cancer can only be made by biopsy of the prostate.

Another potentially helpful parameter in determining if a PSA level is worrisome enough to do a prostate biopsy is finding significant increases in the PSA levels from year to year. Clearly, this can only be helpful if a patient has had at least a couple of prior PSA tests over a period of time. In general, a PSA increase of less than 0.7 unit in one year's time is considered acceptable. Increases of more than this are potentially worrisome even if these increases still leave the patient well within the limits of normal PSA levels. In other words, if the patient had a PSA of 1.2 the last couple of years and it suddenly went to 2.5, this change would, in my opinion, definitely trigger the need for a biopsy of the prostate gland.

Still another attempt to better home in on the significance of PSA elevations as a means to minimize the incidence of negative prostate biopsies (in other words, to attempt to limit as best as possible the use of the prostate biopsy to those patients where the finding of prostate cancer is likely) is the concept of "free PSA" as a blood test for prostate cancer. This concept of free PSA for prostate cancer uses a ratio in which the free PSA (the unbound portion) is the numerator and the total PSA is the denominator. The rationale for this concept of free PSA is that when prostate cells become malignant, the PSA that they produce tends to leak into the blood stream more than the PSA that is produced by benign prostate cells does. For reasons that are not well comprehended, it is a fact that the percentage of this free PSA is lower in patients with prostate cancer than in patients with any benign condition that might elevate the total PSA level. Therefore, in a patient in whom prostate cancer exists, the unbound, or free, PSA level usually is less than 25 percent of the total PSA in the blood as expressed in a ratio of the unbound to total PSA. When the PSA elevation is due to conditions other than cancer, the free PSA is usually more than 25 percent of the total PSA expressed as a ratio of the unbound to total PSA. It is important to realize, however, that this measurement of free PSA is by no means a foolproof means of determining whether a given PSA elevation represents cancer. It is simply another means by which it is hoped that the number of negative prostate biopsies could be reduced.

The technical name for PSA is human kallikrein 3. Researchers in the field are now working with human kallikrein 2 (hK2) in the hope that it will be yet another, and better, means of identifying those patients with elevated PSA levels who do not in fact need prostate biopsies because no cancer is present in the prostate gland. Experimentally, hK2 serum levels have been found to increase in the presence of prostate cancer, and it is hoped that in the future a combination of hK2 levels and the free-to-total PSA ratio may result in eliminating the need for many biopsies of the prostate that turn out to be negative, thereby saving some patient discomfort and anxiety as well as considerable cost. There is one further blood test that is still very very much in the investigational stage, and that is the measurement of complex PSA. This is not simply a mathematical determination of what is left over when the free PSA is subtracted from the total PSA, but rather it is a specific measurement in itself that some investigators have indicated may be helpful in detecting those patients with elevated PSA levels who do indeed have prostate cancer. At the present time, it is not in general clinical usage.

You may have gathered from the foregoing that although PSA is, in my opinion, the best tumor marker in all of medicine, it is not able by itself to either diagnose or refute the presence of prostate cancer. Rather, it very commonly leads a patient to the next step which is a prostate biopsy if the PSA is elevated. This in turn often leads to anxiety for the patient, some discomfort, and considerable expense. Moreover, it has never been documented in a prospective study that the early diagnosis of prostate cancer resulting from PSA testing leads to an increased life expectancy. For these reasons, there are many physicians as well as many professional organizations that feel PSA testing should not be done routinely. I strongly disagree with this but with the caveat that I only recommend it for men who are about 70 years of age or less.

There is no question that all cancers grow and spread and ultimately kill; the questions are how rapidly does a given cancer grow and spread and kill and what are the odds of a patient's dying of something else in the meantime? Since the life expectancy of most prostate cancer patients is about ten years from the time of early diagnosis without any definitive treatment (except delayed hormone treatment ultimately; see Chapter 5), I generally do not recommend specific treatment such as surgery or radiation for a patient who is over 70 years of age who has been diagnosed with prostate cancer. I base this on the fact that life expectancy for most people over 70 years of age is usually at or about ten years. Since I do not usually recommend any definitive treatment (surgery or radiation) for a patient over age 70, I do not usually recommend routine PSA testing either in this age group. On the other hand, if a patient who is older than the early seventies has been diagnosed with prostate cancer and specifically requests definitive treatment, I am perfectly willing to refer him for radiation therapy even though I would not personally consider attempting a curative surgical procedure (a radical prostatectomy) in a man who is over 70.

For younger men, however, particularly those in their forties, fifties, and sixties in whom life expectancies of twenty and more years can fairly be anticipated, I feel that PSA testing is very definitely indicated with follow-up biopsies and treatment as needed. My own rule of thumb is that if a man is an African American or if he is a white man and has a first-degree relative (a father or brother) in whom prostate cancer was diagnosed before the age of 60, I recommend annual PSA testing and a digital rectal exam beginning at age 40. For all other white men, I recommend PSA testing and an annual digital rectal examination beginning at age 50.

A final word about PSA levels and how high they may go. I have seen them as high as 3,000 in patients with widespread and diffusely metastatic prostate cancer involving many bones of the body. In general, if the PSA is under 10, there is probably about a 25 percent chance of prostate cancer being present. The higher it is above this level, the greater the likelihood of prostate cancer. If the PSA is as high as 50 or higher, the likelihood of prostate cancer is great but there is still a good chance that the cancer is confined within the prostate gland although this is by no means certain. Once the PSA has reached a level of about 100 or higher, the odds are great that the cancer has spread well outside the prostate gland.

A final word about prostatic acid phosphatase, a blood test that was the standard in cases of prostate cancer until the advent of PSA testing. I do not believe the prostatic acid phosphatase blood test is of any benefit in determining the presence of early prostate cancer although if it is elevated, it can be helpful in determining that prostate cancer has spread outside the prostate gland and to bone.

X-ray Studies and Other Imaging Techniques

The Excretory Urogram

Sometimes referred to as an IVP, or intravenous pyelogram, this single x-ray study provides the urologist with an extraordinary amount of information about virtually the entire urinary tract. It is performed by injecting into a vein on the forearm a substance that will appear white against the dark background of the x-ray. The white color of the substance within the kidney produces an image on the x-ray film of the kidneys and their interior and then, sequentially, the ureters, the bladder, and the urethra, as the injected substance, mixed with urine, moves in a downward fashion from the kidneys toward the bladder and then toward the outside. Until fairly recently, the substance that was injected so these x-rays could be done not infrequently resulted in nausea, vomiting, itching, rash, and even occasionally very serious reactions including the extremely infrequent fatal reaction.

Unfortunately, it is quite impossible to predict which patients will have either mild or severe reactions since there is virtually nothing in a person's past history that would make the doctor suspicious of an impending problem other than the very obvious statement by a patient that a prior excretory urogram had unpleasant or even serious side effects. More recently, radiologists have been using a nonionic form of contrast to perform excretory urograms, and this has greatly decreased the incidence of the mild reactions although the occasional severe and even fatal reaction does still occur. In patients in whom there is a question about a prior allergic history to any contrast material, a day or two of oral steroids (cortisone) and antihistamines are administered prior to making the x-rays, but whether this offers any real protection against a severe reaction is questionable.

It should go without saying, on the basis of the foregoing, that an excretory urogram because of its inherent albeit very, very slight risk of leading to a serious reaction should only be done when there is a true indication for it.

The excretory urogram, which is a series of films that are exposed over a period of about thirty minutes, is useful for many urologic conditions, and it is primarily used to visualize and examine the kidneys (Fig. 2–1). Its specific relevance to

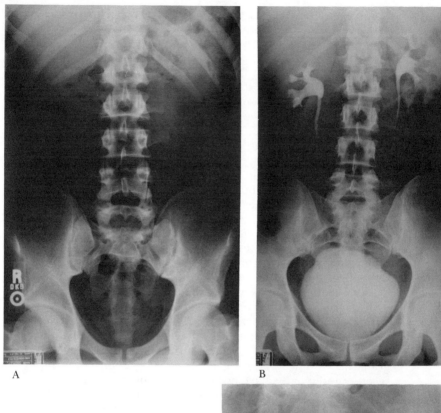

A

B

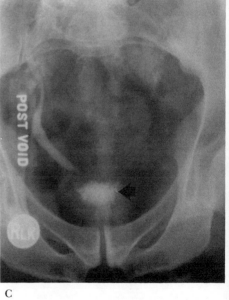

C

diseases of the prostate gland is therefore somewhat limited. Historically, the excretory urogram has been used to estimate how well a patient empties his bladder during voiding as well as to see if there is any obstruction to the drainage of a kidney caused by the enlarged prostate gland. Also, the excretory cystogram phase of the excretory urogram can offer some idea about the size of the prostate gland based on the negative shadow that it casts within the bladder itself. Although many urologists still obtain an excretory urogram prior to any contemplated prostate surgery, I believe that most urologists feel it is not necessary to do this in every situation and that an ultrasound examination of the kidneys as well as an ultrasound examination of the bladder is just as effective in determining whether there is any obstruction to the kidneys and how well the patient is able to empty his bladder. I do feel, however, that for any patient with microscopic or visible blood in the urine, an excretory urogram is the study of choice since it is the preferred test for detecting any possible tumors within the lining of the kidney or the ureters. Assuming that a patient has normal renal function as demonstrated by a normal blood creatinine level, I don't think any specific studies to delineate how well the kidneys are working, such as with a renal scan (see below) or an excretory urogram, are necessary.

For patients with known prostate cancer, an excretory

Figure 2–1   *A. KUB (kidney, ureter, bladder) film. This is the preliminary film that is taken before any contrast material is injected into the patient. It shows the kidney areas, the soft tissue areas through which the ureters travel on their way to the bladder, the bladder area, and all of the bony structures.*

B. X-ray taken some minutes after the injection of the contrast material, showing normal kidneys, ureters, and bladder. Note particularly the appearance of the bladder, which is full and perfectly normal.

C A postvoid film showing an insignificant amount of contrast material left in the bladder (arrow). This film is taken after the patient has been asked to void the urine and contrast material that has accumulated in the bladder and which is seen in panel B. Following voiding, there should be an insignificant amount of contrast material remaining in the bladder.

urogram may be used to demonstrate obstruction to one or both ureters that may occur from the spread of the cancer. However, this knowledge can be gained equally from a renal scan or a renal ultrasound (see below). The initial film of the excretory urogram (Fig. 2–1A) can also often reveal a spread of cancer to one or more of the bones of the pelvis or the spine.

For most patients with infection or inflammation of the prostate gland, an excretory urogram is usually not necessary.

Renal Scans

Renal scanning is yet another method of "visualizing" the urinary tract, but the visualization is done by detecting the radioactivity over the kidneys (using a gamma camera) that results when a radioactive material is injected intravenously. This radioactivity is then seen on a monitor and transferred to a piece of paper rather than to an x-ray film (Fig. 2–2). The radiation exposure from these renal scans comes from a radioactive material that is injected, but the total amount of radiation is much less than that received by the patient when an excretory urogram (IVP) is done since the radiation exposure to the patient having the IVP procedure is from the x-rays themselves. Furthermore, there is no risk of an allergic-type reaction with a renal scan. The study is particularly suited for those patients with less than normal kidney function because the visualization of poorly functioning kidneys when excretory urograms are done is not very satisfactory. When renal scans are done, it is not possible to see the precise anatomic detail within the kidney that is seen with an excretory urogram, but renal scanning is an excellent technique for evaluating the blood flow to the kidneys, how well the kidneys are functioning, and whether there is any obstruction to drainage of the kidneys.

Different radioisotopes are concentrated by different parts of the kidneys. These isotopes emit gamma rays which are detected by a gamma camera and put on film. The emitted gamma rays will have a characteristic pattern that depends on the specific isotope used which in turn depends on the specific cells of the kidney concentrating the isotope. The specific pattern of the emitted gamma rays for a given individual can

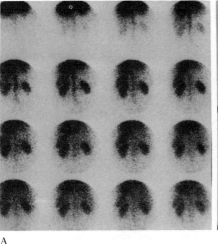

A

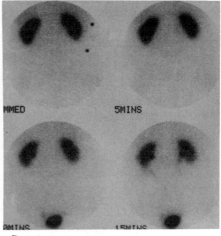

B

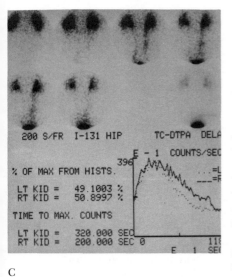

C

Figure 2-2   A NORMAL "TRIPLE" RENAL SCAN

A. The blood flow to the kidneys beginning seconds after the injection of the radioisotope. Each kidney is seen with equal intensity showing equal blood flow to the two kidneys.

B. Two equal, well-functioning kidneys several minutes after injection of the radioisotope. The specific kidney function being measured is the glomerular filtration rate, and it is measured by noting how many minutes it takes following injection of the radioisotope for the radioactivity over the kidneys to reach a maximum.

C. Measuring the second major function of the kidney, known as tubular secretion. This same image also notes the presence or absence of any obstruction to the drainage of the kidneys.

then be compared with known normal patterns for that isotope thereby permitting the interpretation of renal scans as
normal or abnormal. The use of renal scanning in prostatic
diseases is infrequent and certainly not used as often as excretory urography or ultrasonography although it probably
could be used much more frequently as a diagnostic study to
evaluate kidney function and possible kidney obstruction. It
does, however, not provide very much information regarding
the actual anatomy of the kidney.

Ultrasound

This is a totally noninvasive and benign procedure for
which there are literally no risks and no radiation exposure.
The procedure is used to image many different structures
within the body. When combined with renal scanning, it provides virtually as much information about the kidneys (Fig.
2–3) as an excretory urogram does, and it is remarkably adept
at determining whether various masses found within the kidney on the excretory urogram, for example, are cystic or solid
in nature. The principle of ultrasonography is similar to that
of sonar which is a means by which objects underwater (as, for
example, a submarine) may be identified by a ship on the surface of the water. A series of high-frequency sound waves are
generated by the vibration of a crystal within the ultrasound
machine, and the crystal then "listens" for the echo response.
These responses are transmitted as electric signals to a screen
that records and diagrams the signals, and the shape seen on
the screen reflects the shape and consistency of the object
returning the sound waves. Ultrasound in urology is of great
use in examining the kidneys and in discriminating between
the different types of masses that occur commonly in kidneys, particularly in the differentiation between a mass that is
totally cystic (filled with a clear fluid and perfectly benign),
one that is solid (with a good possibility of being cancer),
and one that is both cystic and solid (which may or may not
have cancer within it). For patients with prostate infection or
inflammation, ultrasound is only of minimal benefit in making
a diagnosis and it is used infrequently for patients with these
conditions.

For benign prostatic hyperplasia, ultrasound can be help-

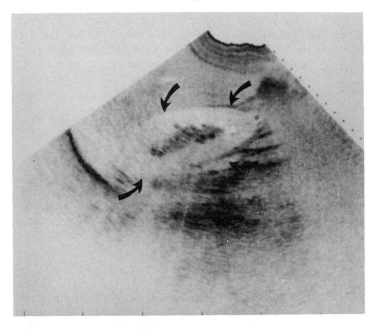

Figure 2–3   *Normal ultrasound of the kidney. Arrows outline the kidney. The dark outline in the center of the kidney is caused by the normal complex structures that are in the center of the kidney.*

ful in estimating the size of the prostate gland in order to determine the best surgical approach to it, since the surgical approach is often guided by the size of the gland. However, there are equally good methods of estimating prostate size that do not require ultrasound. Finally, it should be noted that ultrasound adds nothing at all to the question of *whether* surgery for benign prostatic hyperplasia is indicated (see Chapter 4). The principal use of ultrasound as far as the prostate is concerned is in visualizing the prostate gland for the purpose of obtaining prostatic biopsies in patients for whom biopsy of the prostate is indicated. This would be for those patients having an elevated PSA blood level or having an abnormal digital rectal examination of the prostate or both (see Chapter 4). Ultrasound of the prostate is not indicated for the purpose of screening a patient for possible prostatic cancer, assuming that the patient has a normal PSA blood test and a normal digital rectal examination. However, once biopsies of the prostate are indicated, the use of ultrasound is of great help in assisting the placement of these biopsies so that as much of the prostate gland as possible is sampled. Most prostate cancers will appear as hypoechoic areas on ultrasound (this means areas that are less dense than the surrounding prostate tissue), but it is a fact that most of these hypoechoic areas are not malignant. Nevertheless, any areas seen to be hypoechoic are biopsied after which biopsies of several different areas of the prostate gland are obtained.

The imaging studies that have just been described— excretory urograms, renal scans, and ultrasound—are sometimes done by urologists and sometimes done by radiologists. In the majority of clinical settings in this country, radiologists do the excretory urograms although there are many urologic offices where these studies are performed. The renal scans are mostly done by specialists in nuclear medicine, which is a division of radiology, although some urologists also perform these studies. The ultrasound examinations of the prostate gland are most commonly performed by urologists who do the prostate biopsies at the same time as the ultrasound examination. However, in some centers it is a joint effort between the radiologists who visualize the prostate gland and the urologists who do the biopsies.

Computed Tomography (CT) Scanning

This extraordinary diagnostic tool has been in common use since the late 1970s. It is an imaging method that combines the use of x-ray with computer technology. The computer is able to construct a two-dimensional image of a cross section of the body from data obtained by taking x-rays at 1-centimeter intervals through the part of the body that is being studied. A major advantage of this cross-sectional viewing of the body is being able to see anatomic, and particularly abnormal, findings in an anterior-posterior relationship that would simply not be seen with standard or conventional x-ray techniques. Besides providing this cross-sectional view (standard x-rays offer a longitudinal view), perhaps the greatest advantage of CT scanning over conventional radiography is the ability of these scans to detect differences in density between parts of the body far better than can be done with more conventional x-ray studies. CT scanning is therefore extraordinarily useful in the evaluation of abnormal masses anywhere in the body because these scans are often able to determine whether these masses are dense enough to be suspicious for malignant tumors or are, in fact, benign cystic lesions. Tumors of the kidney are much denser than benign, cystic lesions of the kidney since the latter are usually filled with clear fluid. Moreover, the density of the kidney tumor is different from the adjacent normal kidney tissue. It is sometimes more dense and sometimes less dense, but it is different enough that it provides another means by which a malignancy can be detected.

The major role of CT scanning in urologic diagnosis is in determining the nature of masses within the kidney as well as determining if there is any obvious spread of malignancies from the kidney to other parts of the abdomen or pelvis; the CT scans are also most beneficial in evaluating the presence of cancer that may have spread from the bladder. In terms of the prostate gland, CT scans are of limited use and have virtually no genuine role in the evaluation of infection or inflammation of the prostate or benign prostatic hyperplasia. It is true that some urologists elect to get CT scans of the pelvis in patients with known prostate cancer to see if there is any obvious spread of the prostate cancer prior to initiating any treatment. As a general rule, CT scans are of very limited value in determining the spread of prostate cancer although they are of some benefit in determining if there has been any local extension of the prostate cancer outside of the prostate gland (Fig. 2–4). I personally do not believe that CT scans have a very great role in the management of patients with prostate cancer except, perhaps, in very limited and unique situations.

Magnetic Resonance Imaging (MRI)

This imaging technique is newer than CT scanning and has been in relatively common usage in this country since the mid-1980s. It relies heavily on computer assistance and is somewhat similar to a CT scan in that cross-sectional images can be obtained. However, this versatile but enormously expensive machine can also make images in the longitudinal,

A

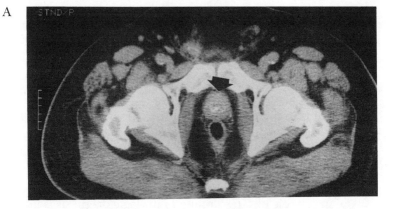

Figure 2–4   A. A CT scan of the pelvis showing a normal prostate
gland (arrow).
    B. A CT scan showing a greatly enlarged prostate with irregular
margins due to a large and extensive prostate cancer (arrows). Both
panels A and B are cross-sectioned through the pelvis.

B

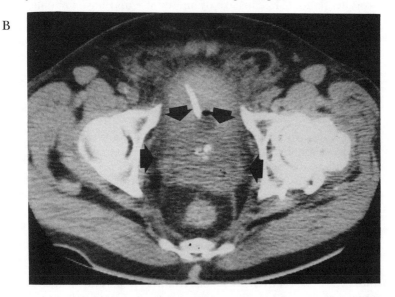

sagittal, and oblique planes. The method of obtaining the image is entirely different from that with CT scanning, and there is one very major improvement over CT scanning: the patient is not exposed to any radiation and there is therefore no known hazard to this study. Further, it is not necessary to introduce any contrast material into the bowel or the kidney in order to do the imaging (Fig. 2–5). The MRI image is seen on a screen and then transferred to photographic film. This MRI modality offers little over CT scanning in trying to determine if there has been any extensive spread from a primary prostate cancer. However, it is somewhat better than CT scanning in trying to determine if there has been any local extension of the prostate cancer beyond the prostate capsule, and for this purpose optimum results are achieved when a coil is placed in the rectum at the time that the MRI scanning is being done. However, MRI scanning is not considered to be a routine part of the diagnostic workup for patients with prostate cancer, and I personally do not use it.

Bone Scanning and Bone X-rays

These are studies that are done when a diagnosis of prostatic cancer has been established or is strongly suspected. These studies are done for the purpose of "staging" the prostatic cancer. *Staging* is a medical term for the process of determining if a known cancer is still confined within the prostate and is therefore probably curable or if it has spread outside the prostate gland and is therefore not curable. One of the most common places to which prostate cancer spreads is to the bones, particularly those of the spine, the hips, the pelvis, and the long bones of the upper leg. When prostate cancer does spread to bone, it damages and even destroys that bone to some degree. As soon as this damage or destruction has occurred, the body's natural healing process begins to lay down new bone in the damaged area.

If x-rays of the damaged bone are taken, the initial appearance is that of a *lytic* lesion, a medical term for the result of the destructive process that gives the bone a thinned-out appearance in the x-ray and makes it look as if it has virtually no substance. As new bone is laid down by the body's natural healing process, it gives an x-ray appearance of the bone that

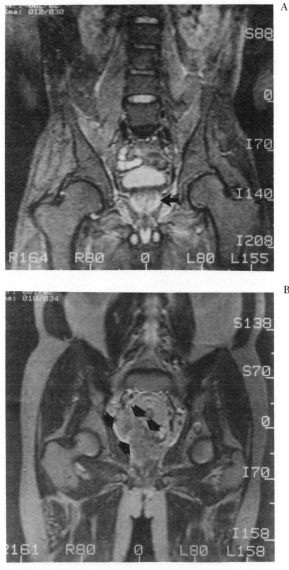

Figure 2–5   MAGNETIC RESONANCE IMAGING (MRI)
   A. A normal prostate gland (arrow).
   B. An extensive cancer of the prostate extending in an upward direction (arrows). Both panels A and B are longitudinal images through the pelvis.

is much denser than normal. This appearance is referred to as *blastic* (Fig. 2–6). Obviously, there is a lag between the time that destruction of the bone begins and the time when it becomes visible on x-ray as either a lytic or blastic lesion.

However, between three and six months before anything at all is visible on an x-ray, the changes that have occurred in bone from a spreading cancer can be visualized by means of bone scans which are much more sensitive at detecting early destruction and repair in bone than are x-rays. These scans are performed by injecting intravenously a radioisotope which moves from the blood into the bone cells that are in a reparative phase. The amount of the radioisotope taken up by the bone is then counted by a device—very similar to a Geiger counter—which counts the amount of radioactivity (from the radioisotope) over the bone and displays each of these counts as a dot on a screen or a monitor. A bone that has a heavy count of radioactivity over it can be readily visualized on the monitor and then on a photographic piece of paper to which it is transferred (Fig. 2–7).

An increased number of counts of radioisotope in one or more bony areas is considered to be strong presumptive evidence of the laying down of new bone which is usually in response to bone destruction. However, it is not proof of the presence of cancer that has spread to bone. Any process that can destroy bone, such as an injury or even arthritis, will result in the initiation of the bone reparative mechanism and this will lead in turn to an increased number of counts of radioactivity over those bony areas. In other words, a "positive" bone scan means only that bony destruction and the reparative process have occurred; it does *not* indicate what caused the bony destruction. However, if the isotope scans are compared with the bone x-rays and the areas of increased uptake are seen to have a perfectly normal appearance on x-ray (as opposed to an appearance of new or old trauma or arthritis), then the probability of metastatic cancer becomes the most likely diagnosis. Note that if the bone x-rays themselves show blastic or lytic lesions, there is usually no need to do a bone scan.

Bone scans are not indicated in the management of patients with benign prostatic hyperplasia or with infection or inflammation of the prostate.

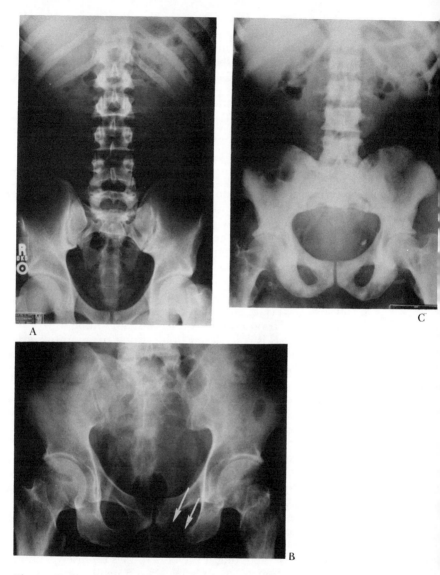

Figure 2–6   A. Normal bone x-rays.
    B. Lytic lesion in the bone (arrows) caused by virtually complete destruction of the bone from the spread of prostate cancer.
    C. Blastic lesions diffusely seen through the spine and pelvis caused by the laying down of new bone secondary to extensive damage from the spread of prostate cancer. These blastic lesions give the bones the appearance of being more dense than normal.

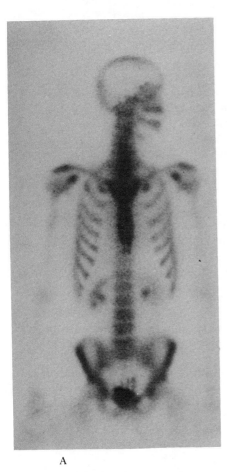
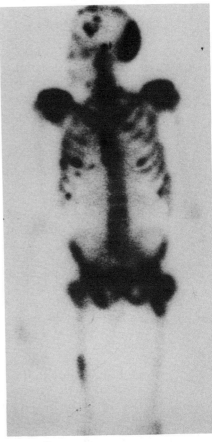

A   B

Figure 2–7   BONE SCANS
   A. A normal bone scan.
   B. A strongly positive bone scan with greatly increased uptake of radioisotope in many bones, particularly the skull, the shoulders, and the pelvis, due to an extensive spread of cancer from the prostate to these bony areas.

Urodynamic Studies

The urinary bladder has two basic functions: urine storage and urine evacuation (voiding). Urodynamic studies are simply tests by which a physician is able to measure these functions as an objective means of evaluating the act of voiding and, more importantly, abnormalities of voiding. These urodynamic studies have many valuable functions in several urologic diseases, but the applicability of these to prostatic disease is predominantly in those patients with benign prostatic hyperplasia. To a much lesser extent, these studies have an occasional role in the evaluation of patients with symptoms of prostatic inflammation (see Chapter 3). Urodynamic studies generally play no role in the evaluation or treatment of patients with prostatic cancer although they may have a very definite role in the management of certain voiding problems that sometimes occur following the surgical treatment of prostatic cancer (see Chapter 8).

Patients with benign prostatic hyperplasia (see Chapter 4) generally have symptoms such as a weak urinary stream, hesitancy in starting the stream, interruption of the stream before voiding has been completed, and even dribbling of urine after voiding has been completed and the trousers have been closed. These symptoms suggest the likelihood of obstruction of the bladder due to the prostate gland. Still other patients with bladder outlet obstruction have symptoms of voiding frequency, particularly at night (nocturia), and urgency with or without urge incontinence. Either of these groups of symptoms most often are associated with bladder outlet obstruction caused by the prostate gland.

However, in a small percentage of cases, these symptoms can be due to causes quite unrelated to the prostate gland. In the case of the first group of symptoms, for instance, a weak bladder muscle, which might be due to diabetes or some neurologic condition, can produce the symptoms of a weak urinary stream—difficulty starting the stream, and so on. Moreover, the aging bladder in both men and women tends to become somewhat overactive thereby producing the symptoms of frequency, urgency, and so on. This overactivity of the bladder can be caused by an obstructing prostate but can also be a primary bladder problem unrelated to any prostatic obstruction. In point of fact, about 80 percent of the time that a man over 50 has any of these symptoms, the cause is obstruction by the prostate gland. However, at least 20 percent of the time the symptoms are not due to prostatic obstruction but to one or more bladder problems. Therefore, I feel it is extremely precipitous and quite unwise to proceed to an interventional (surgical) treatment of presumed prostatic obstruction without being as certain as one can be that this is indeed the cause of the patient's symptoms.

The study that I feel is most helpful in differentiating between an obstructing prostate gland and a primary bladder problem as the cause of these symptoms is the pressure/flow study. In this study, a very small catheter with two channels running through it is placed into the patient's bladder. One of these channels is connected to a machine that measures bladder pressures when the bladder is filling through the other channel, when the bladder is full, and when the patient then begins to void on demand around this very small catheter. At the time of this voiding, the rate of urine flow in cubic centimeters per second is measured using a device for this purpose. The software in the machine itself is then able to set up a nomogram using the bladder pressure at the time of voiding and the rate of flow at the time of voiding and is, to a very great degree, thereby able to tell the examining urologist whether obstruction to the flow of urine does in fact exist.

My own rule of thumb is that if the bladder pressure is 50–60 centimeters of water or higher and the maximum urine flow rate is less than 10 cubic centimeters per second, obstruction exists. Alternatively, if the bladder pressure at the time of voiding is over 100 centimeters of water regardless of the rate of flow of urine at the time of voiding, obstruction is also said to exist. It is important to realize, however, that the bladder pressures referred to must be those achieved by the bladder during the natural act of voiding (or attempted voiding) and must not reflect pressure within the bladder when the patient is using his abdominal muscles to push or strain in an attempt to void as this will artificially increase bladder pressure. It also must not include bladder pressures noted during bladder filling which are involuntary and not related to voiding attempts (an overactive bladder).

This pressure/flow study can also diagnose the cause of symptoms such as frequency and urgency when the bladder pressure and flow rate are within normal limits but the pressure within the bladder as the bladder fills tends to "spike" inappropriately thereby indicating an overactive bladder. Normally, bladder pressure during filling increases only very very slightly until the bladder capacity has been reached; however, in patients with an overactive bladder, there will be involuntary spikes representing increased bladder pressure that occurs inappropriately. By means of this pressure/flow study, therefore, the urologist is best able to predict those patients who will achieve the best results from surgical intervention. Obviously, if pharmacologic treatment of a patient's symptoms is to be used instead of surgical treatment, it is not necessary to do this pressure/flow study initially because there is very little lost if this type of drug therapy does not work.

The equipment necessary to do these pressure/flow studies is expensive (Fig. 2–8) and is not necessarily found in every urologic office. One of the reasons for the great expense of this equipment is that in addition to the means of diagnosing pressures within the bladder and urinary flow rates, it can also include a fluoroscope. It is often quite helpful to obtain a fluoroscopic image during the act of voiding because this enables the urologist to specifically see where the point of obstruction may be. This fluoroscopy can be very costly for the patient, however. Although I do not feel this fluoroscopy is necessary in all or even most cases where one is evaluating presumed bladder outlet obstruction, it is helpful at times, but it does certainly add to the cost of the equipment and of the procedure. As noted, there are many urologists who feel it is not necessary to do these studies prior to a surgical intervention for what is presumed to be bladder outlet obstruction, and, in general, this is true in the majority of cases. However, I prefer to do these studies in virtually all patients in whom surgery for prostatic obstruction is considered, for the reasons already given.

Bladder Catheterization

Two distinct types of bladder catheterization are carried out and two distinct types of catheter are used (Fig. 2–9). One type is the "in-and-out" catheterization in which, for example, the catheter is put into the bladder for a very brief period of time in order to measure the amount of residual urine immediately following voiding, an amount which is normally near 0 milliliters. I should mention here in passing that although this

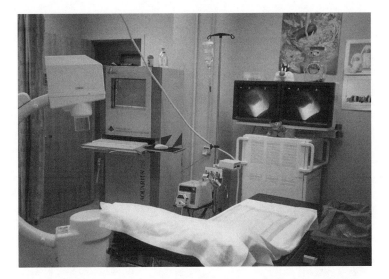

Figure 2–8   *A state-of-the-art setup for performing urodynamic studies. Specifically, this type of equipment is used to measure pressure/flow studies as described in the text. Note that the capability for cine fluoroscopy is included with this equipment; this is sometimes used along with pressure/flow studies to pinpoint the precise location of an obstruction.*

is certainly the most precise measurement of urine that is left behind following voiding, it is not used very frequently since this amount of postvoid residual urine can be measured with reasonable accuracy using ultrasound equipment which is noninvasive and certainly much more comfortable for the patient. In any case, when benign prostatic hyperplasia obstructs the bladder outlet, incomplete bladder emptying will usually occur eventually, and the larger the amounts of residual urine left following voiding, the more important it is to treat and relieve the obstruction. This in-and-out catheterization may be done intermittently several times a day for individuals who are unable to empty their bladder adequately whether the cause of the inability to empty the bladder is an obstructing prostate or a nerve deficiency to the bladder such as may occur with diabetes or after an injury to the spinal cord. Such nerve deficiencies may render the bladder quite incapable of its normal function. In-and-out catheterization

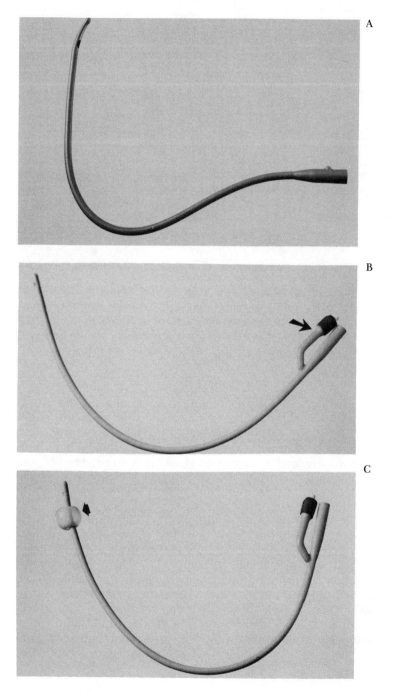

A

B

C

may also be used to instill solutions into the bladder such as a contrast medium for x-ray purposes or various medications for certain kinds of bladder disease.

The second broad category of catheterization is done with a special type of catheter which is then left indwelling within the bladder for varying periods of time. This type of catheter, known as a Foley, is able to stay inside the bladder because of a bag on its end that is inflated once the catheter is within the bladder thereby preventing the catheter from falling out. Long-term catheter drainage of this sort may be done for many different reasons, but for patients with prostatic enlargement it is done to facilitate continuous emptying of the bladder in individuals who are either totally unable to void because of the obstructing prostate tissue or who void so inefficiently that they leave behind large amounts of residual urine. As a general rule, the indwelling catheter for these patients is left in place only until surgical correction of the obstructing prostate tissue can be carried out. In such patients in-and-out catheterization is preferable to leaving a Foley catheter in place, but there are some individuals who feel that they are not able to perform this catheterization procedure and who prefer to have the Foley catheter left in place. Rarely, continuous catheter drainage (or indefinite in-and-out drainage) may continue indefinitely in a patient who refuses surgical treatment or whose general medical condition is so bad that he is not considered a suitable risk for surgery or who just plain prefers to continue with catheter drainage.

As a urologist, I rarely think twice about catheterizing a

Figure 2–9   CATHETERS USED TO DRAIN THE BLADDER
A. A straight catheter, which is used for "in-and-out" catheterization.

B. A Foley catheter, which is used when the catheter is to be left in the bladder for a period of time. The arrow points to the side arm on the catheter, through which a bag on the other end of the catheter is inflated. The other portion of the catheter adjacent to the arrow is that part of the catheter through which urine drains, usually into a collecting bag.

C. A Foley catheter with the bag on the end inflated (arrow). It is inflated after it has been placed inside the bladder, and the inflated bag catches on the inside of the bladder neck, thereby preventing the catheter from falling out.

patient when I feel it is in his best interest. Catheterization is a procedure that is so commonly and frequently done, by virtually all physicians, that I sometimes tend to overlook the extreme apprehension that can be brought on by the very *thought* of catheterization. I realize that when a catheterization is done, it is neither painful nor harmful, but I am also a man and can therefore understand the anxieties and concerns about an invasion of that most holy of holy parts of the male body. When a catheterization is necessary, whether it is in my office or the hospital, I make a point of always explaining to my patient exactly what the procedure entails. Furthermore, I show him a catheter, exactly like the one that will be used, and tell him that the opening inside his penis is much, much larger than the catheter and therefore the procedure cannot possibly hurt him. I do, however, tell my patients that they may well find the procedure to be unpleasant. I have been catheterized myself and I tell this to my patients. I further tell them that the experience was far more unpleasant in contemplation than in the execution which was not at all painful but which was mentally distressing simply because of the *thought* of what was being done to me. When I show the catheter to a patient, I make a point of having him feel it so he can realize that it truly is made of soft rubber. I am convinced that this additional time spent with my patient prior to catheterization is time very well spent. When it is a Foley indwelling that is being used, I will show my patients exactly how the bag on the end of the catheter is inflated and then deflated when it is to be removed and explain that neither of these acts will cause them any discomfort nor will removing the catheter when it is no longer needed. In actual fact, I do not think I can remember having a patient who has been properly prepared tell me that a catheterization, carefully done and using lots of lubricating jelly, has been painful or distressing or really anything worse than a less-than-pleasant experience.

Cystoscopy

The diagnostic procedure that is most frequently associated with the specialty of urology and with urologic disease is undoubtedly the cystoscopic examination of the bladder and the urethra. This examination is virtually the exclusive domain of urologists, and the precise and detailed knowledge obtained from it is but one example of how diagnostic techniques help to make urology the accurate and precise specialty that it is.

Cystoscopy involves the passage of a hollow instrument with a light and a lens on one end and a viewing lens on the other into the penile urethra and then into the bladder. Through the hollow instrument, urine that is in the bladder can run to the outside, thereby enabling the measurement of the urine that is in the bladder, and this can be considered a fairly accurate measurement of postvoid residual urine if the patient has voided immediately prior to cystoscopy. Once the bladder has been emptied of its contents, water is allowed to flow by gravity through the cystoscope *into* the bladder. This is necessary in order to inflate the bladder away from the lens end of the cystoscope. For example, if you were to put your head inside a balloon, you would have to inflate the balloon away from your eye in order to adequately visualize the interior of the balloon; for the same reason, the bladder must be inflated away from the cystoscope lens. Once the bladder has been filled, it is possible to visualize with detail and accuracy the interior of the bladder. When visualizing the inside of the prostate gland and the inside of the urethra, it is not necessary to have the bladder inflated, because the inside of the prostate and the urethra are tubular in shape and more or less rigid whereas the bladder is a floppy structure that would simply collapse around the lens if it were not inflated.

Cystoscopes have historically been rigid instruments (Fig. 2–10A), but within the past few years flexible cystoscopes have come into common usage (Fig. 2–10B). The passage of these newer, flexible cystoscopes into the bladder is quite similar to the passing of a catheter through the urethra and into the bladder. With either instrument an anesthetic jelly is squirted into the urethra prior to passing the cystoscope. This sufficiently numbs the urethra so patient discomfort is minimal, and the discomfort is actually much more mental than physical. I have always asked male patients after a cystoscopic exam with either instrument how painful it was, and invariably it has been that the thought of what was being done was far more unpleasant than the procedure itself. Whether it is mental or physical, the discomfort is undoubtedly minimized to a certain degree when the flexible cystoscope is used instead of the rigid one.

By using a cystoscope, the urologist is able to visualize the prostatic urethra and to diagnose inflammation of this area

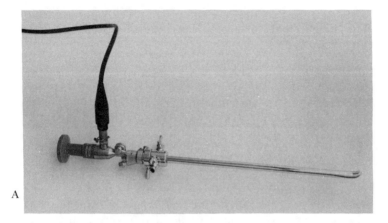

A

Figure 2–10　*A. The standard cystoscope, which is passed through the urethra and is used for visualizing the interior of the bladder and urethra. The black object attached to the cystoscope is the light cord.*

B. The newer and perhaps more frequently used cystoscope is this flexible cystoscope, which serves the same purpose as the standard cystoscope but may be less uncomfortable for the patient because of its flexibility. Note that only the small, curved portion of the cystoscope (arrows) is introduced into the bladder. The light cord is seen leaving the cystoscope at the upper left.

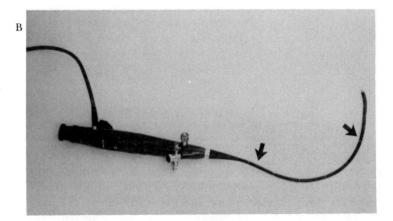

B

such as might be seen with nonspecific urethritis (see Chapter 3). When a diagnosis of benign prostatic hyperplasia (BPH) is being considered (see Chapter 4), cystoscopy may enable the urologist to evaluate and assess the anatomic degree of obstruction caused by the prostate gland and to estimate the size and weight of the obstructing prostate tissue. This enables the urologist to better determine which type of therapeutic approach to use in treating the condition. I would emphasize here, however, that cystoscopy alone cannot make a diagnosis of bladder outlet obstruction other than what appears to be anatomically obstructing. The proper method for diagnosing obstruction has to be based on physiologic function, and it is for this purpose that the pressure/flow study just discussed is carried out. In patients with prostatic cancer, cystoscopy is used to locate sources of prostatic or bladder bleeding that tend to occur with this condition, particularly if the patient's prostate cancer has been treated with radiation therapy.

It is perfectly natural for a man to be extremely apprehensive on learning that he needs to be cystoscoped. This is partly because of anxiety over the unknown, but it is perhaps even more so because of the invasion of the sacred part of the male identity. A thoughtful physician is fully cognizant of this and exerts every effort to make the procedure as nonthreatening as possible and to make the patient as comfortable as possible. Occasionally, if the patient is not going to be driving a car right afterward, an intravenous injection of a tranquilizing or hypnotic agent prior to cystoscopy is helpful, but in my experience this is not usually necessary. I have very rarely used anything more than the requisite local anesthetic jelly instilled into the urethra along with a lot of reassurance and gentleness. The number of patients whom I have encountered over the years who have been unable to tolerate the procedure or who have said afterward that they wished they had been put to sleep or given an injection have been few and far between and have numbered well under 1 percent of all patients.

Prostatic Biopsies

This diagnostic procedure is carried out whenever carcinoma of the prostate is suspected, and it must be noted that prostatic carcinoma can *only* be diagnosed by sampling tissue

from the prostate gland. The suspicion of prostate cancer may
be triggered by several things, but far and away the single
most common finding that arouses the suspicion of prostate
carcinoma is an elevated PSA blood test. Another finding that
can trigger a prostatic biopsy is an abnormal digital rectal
examination of the prostate gland wherein your physician
notes an area of the prostate that is much firmer than the surrounding gland (Fig. 2–11). Sometimes, your physician may
be suspicious of carcinoma simply because of an asymmetric
enlargement of your prostate gland although asymmetry in
and of itself is not often associated with prostate cancer.

Suspicion of cancer should also be aroused when a patient
gives a history of bladder outlet obstruction which sounds
suggestive of benign prostatic hyperplasia but in which the
duration of symptoms is very brief, perhaps three to six
months or even less. Inasmuch as the typical patient with BPH
will have had his symptoms for several years prior to seeing
the physician, a relatively sudden onset of symptoms of blad-

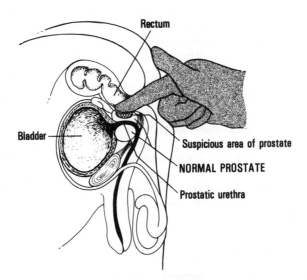

Figure 2–11 *The examining finger in the rectum feeling a hard
or suspicious area of the prostate gland.*

der outlet obstruction should alert the physician to the possibility of a rapidly growing carcinoma of the prostate that is encroaching on and obstructing the prostatic urethra regardless of the feel of the prostate on digital rectal examination. In such cases, but not always, the PSA would be elevated, but it should also be remembered that extremely malignant cancer cells do not necessarily make a great deal of PSA and therefore the PSA level may not be particularly elevated. This is because extremely malignant prostate cancer cells are relatively undifferentiated cells; that is, they do not have the characteristics of prostate cells and hence are unable to make PSA.

Finally, suspicion of prostate cancer should be aroused when a patient visits his physician because of severe pain in one or more bones that has been present for several weeks or longer and has follow-up bone x-rays and/or bone scans that suggest the possibility of bone destruction from some sort of cancer. In the search for the origin of the cancer that has spread to the bone, the prostate must always be high on the suspect list. The alert physician may recommend prostatic biopsy even if the prostate has a relatively normal feel to it.

The prostatic biopsy itself is most often carried out using what is known as a "tru-cut" biopsy needle that is attached to a biopsy gun, and the procedure is almost universally done under ultrasound control. The tru-cut needle (Fig. 2–12) has a hollow end in which the prostate tissue is trapped, and the needle is delivered into the prostate gland using a biopsy "gun" (Fig. 2–13) with such great rapidity that the patient feels virtually no pain. Patients report that these biopsies feel very much like injections and the most uncomfortable part of the procedure is having the ultrasound probe in the rectum.

When visualized on the ultrasound equipment screen, most cancers of the prostate appear less dense than surrounding areas of the prostate (Fig. 2–14). It should be noted that most of these areas that are less dense than the surrounding areas are not necessarily cancer. When the biopsy needle is propelled into the prostate, it is well visualized on the ultrasound screen (Fig. 2–15), and to maximize the likelihood of finding any prostate cancer (if cancer is indeed present in the prostate gland), multiple biopsies are obtained. Traditionally, urologists have biopsied any of these less dense areas in addition to sampling the tissues throughout each side of the prostate gland from the base to the apex. This resulted

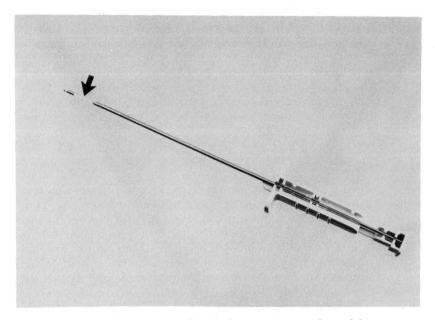

Figure 2–12 *The tru-cut needle, which is most commonly used for prostate biopsies. A core or plug of prostate tissue is obtained within the hollow portion (arrow) of this needle.*

in "sextant" (six in all) biopsies, but the trend now is to obtain even more biopsies particularly from the far lateral reaches of the prostate gland so that nine and often twelve biopsies are often obtained. In this manner, the likelihood of missing any cancer that might be present is diminished.

Prostate biopsy is not indicated for the patient considered to have benign prostatic hyperplasia or for the patient with inflammation or infection in the prostate gland.

Following prostate biopsy, it is not rare to have some blood appear in the urine or in the semen during ejaculation. This simply means that the biopsy needle entered the inside of the prostatic urethra during the course of the biopsy. It is not a cause for worry or alarm. The bleeding will usually stop after a day or two, but if it is heavy or lasts beyond a couple of days, you should tell your urologist. Blood in the semen may last for a number of ejaculations because each time you ejaculate you

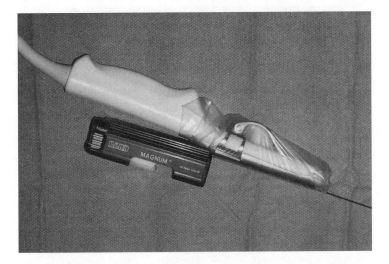

Figure 2–13   *The ultrasound probe, about 2 or 3 inches of which (on the right side of the photo) is inserted into the rectum and over the prostate gland. The tru-cut biopsy needle may be seen extending beyond the tip of this probe, and it is attached to the Magnum biopsy gun, which is spring loaded and fires the needle rapidly into the prostate once the area to be biopsied has been identified using the ultrasound probe. Between six and twelve biopsies of the prostate gland area can be obtained using this equipment.*

cause a violent spasm of the muscles inside your urethra (this is what propels the semen to the outside). This spasm can cause the bleeding to recur before the area is finally healed. If you see blood in the ejaculate, it is probably best to avoid ejaculation for several days in order to let the affected parts heal.

Because a prostate biopsy is carried out through the rectum and because fecal bacteria in the rectum can lead to the introduction of these bacteria into the prostate gland with resulting prostatic infection, every effort is made to clean the rectum as well as possible prior to doing the biopsy. This is done with laxatives taken the night before and an enema on the morning of the biopsy. Additionally, oral antibiotics are given the night before the biopsy, the morning of the biopsy, that evening, and sometimes the following morning as well to minimize even further the chance of resulting prostatic infection.

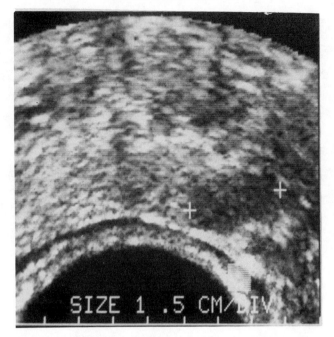

Figure 2-14   *An ultrasound image of the prostate gland. Note the area at the bottom right that is between the two small cross marks. This area is less dense than the surrounding portion of the prostate gland. It is an area such as this that is felt to possibly have cancer within it and which would therefore be biopsied. (Photograph courtesy of Brüel and Kaer Instruments, Inc., Marlborough, Massachusetts.)*

Interpretation of the Prostate Biopsy

Once the biopsy has been done, the obvious question to be answered is is cancer present? Beyond this, and of great importance as far as being one of several factors in predicting success of therapy, is what is the microscopic appearance of the cancer? Is it high grade (very malignant) or relatively low grade (less malignant)? One very common method that pathologists use to determine and report this is a Gleason scale. Using this method, the pathologist grades the cancer as seen on a 1-to-5 scale of increasing malignancy and grades separately both the predominant cancer pattern and the can-

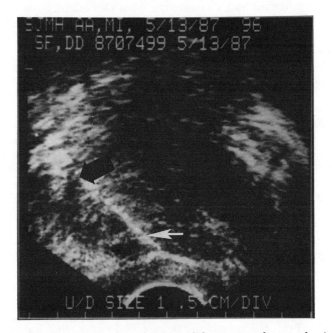

Figure 2–15 *An ultrasound image of the prostate done at the time the prostate biopsies are being taken, showing a biopsy needle (white arrow) within the prostate gland. This biopsy needle appears as a straight-line white area in the lower left portion of the photograph. The tip of the needle is obtaining a biopsy from within a less dense area of the prostate (black arrow) that may possibly have cancer within it. (Photograph courtesy of Brüel and Kaer Instruments, Inc., Marlborough, Massachusetts.)*

cer pattern that appears to be secondary (often these will be the same). These two numbers (each based on a 1-to-5 scale) are then noted and added together to give the Gleason sum, for example, 3 + 3, or 6. Sums of 2, 3, and 4 are considered low-grade (less malignant) cancer; sums of 5, 6, and 7 are of intermediate malignancy, and sums of 8, 9, and 10 are highly malignant. Some pathologists choose to report biopsies simply as grade I (Gleason 2, 3, 4), grade II (Gleason 5, 6, 7), or grade III (Gleason 8, 9, 10). Still other pathologists, although relatively few, prefer to use a 1-to-4 scale with 1's being the least malignant and 4's being the most malignant. Sometimes, the pathologist will report a condition known as Prostatic Intraepithelial Neoplasia (PIN). Prostatic Intraepithelial Neoplasia is reported as low grade or high grade, and it should be noted that high-grade PIN is generally considered to be a premalignant condition. Where this is reported, even in the absence of any definite cancers, repeat biopsies in the very near future are generally indicated because so many of these high-grade PINs do foretell the presence of prostate cancer.

A special situation in which detection of prostate cancer can be much more difficult is that in which a man has had surgery on his intestinal tract and is left with no rectum at all. In this case it is obviously impossible to do a digital rectal exam in order to feel the prostate gland, and so the early suspicion and detection of prostate cancer must be based solely on the PSA blood level. If this level is such that your doctor is concerned about the possibility of prostate cancer, she or he can request that a radiologist obtain a CT scan of your lower abdomen, and at the time that this is done the radiologist may be able to guide a series of needle biopsies of your prostate using the CT image to control the biopsy needle. This is by no means a very satisfactory means of obtaining prostate biopsies; it is difficult to do with any degree of accuracy and it certainly is not always successful. But it is certainly the best that can be achieved under these circumstances.

3

Infection and Inflammation in the Prostate Gland and the Prostatic Urethra, and the Chronic Pelvic Pain Syndrome

A 31-year-old architect came to my office recently in an obvious state of extreme mental anguish. He had called my office earlier that day and been told that I had no available time in my schedule until later in the week. He pleaded with my office secretary to allow him to come in that very day, saying that it was extremely urgent and all but telling her that it was a matter of life or death.

When I saw him later that same afternoon, he was clearly distraught, but he was in no particular pain or discomfort and he appeared to be in excellent health.

"Doctor," he started out, "something is very wrong, and I am frankly scared stiff because of what might happen because of it."

It didn't take me very long to find out that this man had two symptoms and a lot of resulting worry. First, he had noticed a dime-sized brownish stain inside his shorts when he undressed before retiring the previous night. Second, he noticed that the opening at the end of his penis seemed to be glued into a shut position when he woke up that morning. When he pulled apart the two sides of this opening, he noticed a tiny drop of very clear fluid just inside. He had no pain, no discomfort on voiding, did not feel sick, and maintained his usual state of good health. Regardless, he became quite frantic and remained so until his visit to my office. His fear centered around the perceived complications that could result from these two minor symptoms. He was specifically worried that he might develop cancer of the prostate or benign prostatic hyperplasia, but his most severe concern was that his present problem could lead to impotence. This patient was unmarried and had a moderately active sex life compatible with the great time demands of his profession. He had never had anything like this before, he said.

This man's symptoms and problems are common. Indeed, it has been my experience that there is probably no other single group of genitourinary tract symptoms that brings so many male patients to the urologist, and probably to the primary care physician as well, as those that are related to the prostatic urethra and probably to the prostate also. With some exceptions, these different disorders tend to produce rather similar symptoms—with many variations—and it is not an exaggeration to state that there is no other group of disorders, real or imagined, to which young and middle-aged males fall prey that causes more worry, anxiety, and concern than these ailments. In this particular example, my patient had a very mild infection in the prostatic urethra or possibly in his anterior urethra. His anguish well reflects the fact that the concerns and the anxiety that develop in these patients are enormously out of proportion to the severity of the illness and equally out of proportion to the severity of the symptoms. I love to make the analogy between a minimal discharge from the urethra or even an itch or some discomfort in the urethra on the one hand, and a runny nose or an itchy or sore throat on the other. The latter group of symptoms could be present for months or even years without resulting in a patient's visiting his physician, but the former group of symptoms need only be present for a few hours before a very worried and frightened patient comes running to a physician!

A 36-year-old engineer recently came to my office and told me that intermittently for the past three or four years he has had pain in his perineum, pain in his suprapubic area, pain following ejaculation, and frequency of urination. He has not had all of these symptoms at any one time, and there have been times when he has had none of these symptoms. He also told me that to his best knowledge he has never been found to have bacteria in his urine, but he has been on one antibiotic medication or another off and on for the past three years and he estimates that his total time on antibiotic therapy has been about one year. Antibiotics, he says, sometimes make some of his symptoms better but they always recur. He was told by the first urologist that he saw a long time ago that he had "prostatitis," and this was on the basis of the history that he gave to the urologist as well as a digital rectal examination in which the urologist pronounced that the prostate gland felt "boggy."

It is extremely unlikely that this second patient suffers from prostatitis if that term is meant to represent an infection in the prostate gland. The absence of any bacterial infection in the bladder urine pretty well precludes a chronic (or an acute) bacterial infection in the prostate gland if the urine is collected at the time that the patient is having his symptoms. The finding of a "boggy" prostate on digital rectal exam is not related to any pathologic state within the prostate but rather to the frequency of ejaculation. As noted in Chapter 1, a principal function of the prostate gland is to produce and then expel to the outside of the body during ejaculation the fluid in which the spermatozoa travel. If a man has frequent and regular ejaculations, his prostate gland will be relatively firm. On the other hand, if he has not ejaculated in a considerable length of time or if his usual ejaculatory pattern has been sharply decreased, the prostate gland will be full of prostatic fluid and it will feel "boggy" on digital rectal exam. Neither of these digital rectal exam findings should be considered pathologic or indicative of a diseased state.

However, there is a respected school of thought among urologists that feels that the symptoms described by the patient can indeed be related to a "full" prostate resulting from a sudden diminution in ejaculatory frequency such as might be caused by a divorce, a separation, or an illness of the patient's mate. This "full" prostate could indeed be described as "boggy" although certainly not considered indicative of a diseased state. It is sometimes known as "prostatostasis," and it undoubtedly can be responsible for some of the symptoms already noted. This condition is also known as "nonbacterial prostatitis." It may often be treated with some measure of success by increasing the frequency of ejaculation or by frequent and repeated prostatic massages, both of which serve the purpose of emptying the prostate gland.

In the author's experience, however, patients with any or

all of the complaints that primarily consist of perineal or suprapubic pain, postejaculatory pain, or a general feeling of discomfort "deep inside" often suffer from what is now known as "chronic pelvic pain syndrome." This is the new term to encompass the body of symptoms noted here, and it was adopted by a National Institutes of Health (NIH) Consensus Conference held in the mid-1990s. This body of symptoms was so named because it was felt that the majority of times that men had these complaints, they were not caused by the prostate gland at all. Further, by telling a man that he has prostatitis, it is very easy to quite literally make a prostate cripple out of an otherwise normal man, something that would not result if he were simply told that his symptoms were part of a chronic pelvic pain syndrome. It was the feeling of this NIH Consensus Conference that more often than not this chronic pelvic pain syndrome was related to muscle spasms and muscle aches in the pelvic floor (the area that is inside that part of the body which is between the anus and the scrotum). This conclusion was based on several observed facts. First, hundreds of prostate biopsies (done in connection with other studies) showed evidence of chronic inflammation in the prostate gland in patients who had absolutely no symptoms at all referable to the prostate. Second, digital rectal exams when "prostate patients" were having their symptoms would reveal pronounced spasm of these pelvic floor muscles, and third, biofeedback techniques and physical therapy procedures have often had salutary effects for these people.

Recognizing then that there are indeed several conditions which can cause these symptoms and which can be related to the prostate gland and surrounding areas, it becomes necessary to try to differentiate these different conditions. The conditions are infection in the prostatic urethra (the first patient in this chapter), inflammation in the prostate gland in the absence of infection or the chronic pelvic pain syndrome (the second patient noted in this chapter), chronic bacterial infection in the prostate gland (with symptoms very, very similar to the second patient noted), and acute bacterial infection of the prostate gland. Please note that the differentiation between these various conditions is not a haphazard one but may be determined with a reasonable degree of certainty by means of a study described in the next section. Also, it should be noted that if a patient has a chronic bacterial infection in the prostate, the overwhelming likelihood is that he will have bacterial infection in the urine at the time that he is symptomatic.

Diagnostic Studies Used to Differentiate between Inflammation in the Prostatic Urethra, Chronic Bacterial Prostatitis, Chronic Nonbacterial Prostatitis, and Chronic Pelvic Pain Syndrome

When a patient has some—any or all—of the symptoms noted so far in this chapter, it is important to distinguish between the different conditions that can cause the symptoms, and it is particularly important not to tell the patient that he has prostatitis unless this can be documented with reasonable certainty. If there is a discharge from the urethra, however slight, the odds are pretty good that the patient has a nonspecific (posterior) urethritis (inflammation in the prostatic urethra). If the patient's predominant symptoms are perineal pain, pain "deep inside," postejaculatory pain, or even suprapubic pain, the odds are pretty good that he is suffering from what is now known as chronic pelvic pain syndrome, although he may have a nonbacterial inflammation of his prostate gland (prostatostasis). The odds of his having a chronic bacterial prostatitis are very slight since this condition is quite uncommon. Nevertheless, making the correct diagnosis is a matter not so much of playing the odds but rather of attempting to be quite accurate in arriving at a diagnosis, and in my experience, this is something that is rarely done by physicians. Indeed, physical examination is of limited help in differentiating these conditions, and I particularly condemn the practice of doing a digital rectal exam of a prostate, calling it "boggy," and then telling the patient that he therefore has prostatitis. As already noted, the relationship of a "boggy" prostate and a diseased state within the prostate is a very tenuous one indeed! In my opinion, all patients having any, some, or all of the symptoms under discussion should properly have a bacterial localization test which will enable the physician, with reasonable certainty, to determine whether there is any infection in the prostate gland, the urethra, or, as is much more frequently the case, nowhere at all (Fig. 3–1). Note that

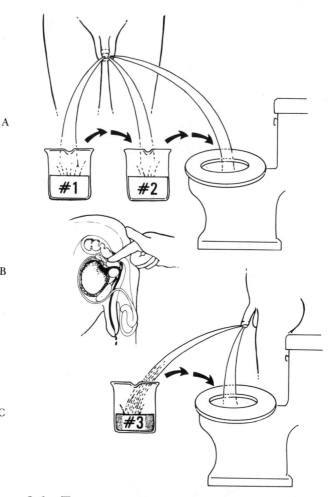

Figure 3–1 TECHNIQUE FOR LOCALIZING THE SOURCE OF
INFECTION TO THE URETHRA OR TO THE PROSTATE

*A. This illustrates the patient starting his urinary stream in
glass #1, continuing it in glass #2 (midstream urine), and finishing it in the toilet, leaving some urine remaining in the bladder.*

*B. This shows the prostate being massaged, or "stripped," by the
physician. Note a drop or two of prostatic secretions coming out of
the penile urethra (something that does not always occur following
prostatic massage).*

*C. This shows glass #3, which represents the first ounce or two
of voiding immediately following the prostatic massage. Glass #3
will contain most of the secretions from the prostate gland. The
patient then finishes voiding into the toilet.*

infection (usually caused by bacteria) is often accompanied by inflammation, but inflammation can be present without any infection.

The patient is asked to begin urinating into a glass marked #1; then, without interrupting his stream, he is asked to void a couple of ounces into the toilet and then a couple of ounces into a glass marked #2; then, again without interrupting his stream, he can void into the toilet while consciously retaining some urine in his bladder. The physician then vigorously massages ("strips") the prostate gland to force prostatic fluid (secretions) out of the prostate gland and into the prostatic urethra. This vigorous massage, or stripping, of the prostate gland is not a painful procedure but it is not a pleasant one either! The discomfort that it may cause varies greatly from patient to patient because the sensitivity of the prostate gland to touch will also vary greatly from patient to patient. The prostatic stripping is done with the patient bent sharply at the waist and leaning over a table so that the physician can easily insert his finger into the rectum. The physician then places his finger on one side of the prostate gland and rolls his finger inward pressing very firmly downward as he rolls his finger from the outside margin of the prostate gland toward the middle of the prostate gland. The physician then moves his finger to the outside margin on the other side of the prostate gland and does the same thing. Each of the two sides of the prostate gland is thus massaged, or stripped, about ten or twelve times. This downward pressure by the physician's finger serves to squeeze the fluid that is normally in the prostate gland out through the various prostatic ducts and into the middle of the prostatic urethra where it pools.

While the prostatic massaging, or stripping, is being done, the patient will often feel that fluid is trying to come out of his penis; this sensation is caused by the prostatic fluid (secretions) pooling in the prostatic urethra. The patient should keep his urethra squeezed shut with his hand during the prostatic massage. At the end of the prostatic massage, these expressed prostatic secretions may travel down the urethra and through the opening at the end of the penis where they are then collected for culture. Usually, however, the prostatic secretions do not leave the penis but remain pooled in the prostatic urethra, and the patient is again asked to begin to urinate after the stripping of the prostate is complete. He is told to void an ounce or two into a glass marked #3. He is then allowed to finish emptying his bladder into the toilet. Glass #3, or the actual prostatic secretions if they come out of the opening in the end of the penis, represent secretions from the interior of the prostate gland. A definitive diagnosis of chronic bacterial prostatitis can then be made if there is at least a tenfold increase in the bacteria colony count obtained from the urine in glass #3 as compared with glass #1, while the culture of urine in glass #2 (the midstream specimen) is sterile.

The bacterial counts for which one is searching in this localization test are in the neighborhood of a few hundred to a few thousand colonies of bacteria per milliliter of urine. A positive test for chronic bacterial prostatitis shows something like 3,000 colonies of bacteria in glass #3 and 300 colonies of bacteria in glass #1. If the bacterial colony count is the same in glass #1 as in glass #3 or if the colony count is greater in glass #1 than in glass #3, then the likely diagnosis is a non-specific urethritis (inflammation in the prostatic urethra). Most frequently, in my experience, there are no bacteria found in any of the specimens, thereby eliminating the diagnosis of chronic bacterial prostatitis or nonspecific urethritis and leaving as the most probable diagnosis that of either chronic nonbacterial prostatitis (prostatostasis) or, much more frequently, chronic pelvic pain syndrome.

To sum up, it is my opinion that it is quite erroneous for a physician to tell a patient that he has a bacterial infection in the prostate gland (chronic bacterial prostatitis) unless either the bacterial colony count in glass #3 exceeds the colony count in glass #1 by a factor of at least ten or the expressed prostatic secretions yield a positive bacterial culture with a colony count tenfold higher than the colony count in glass #1.

Should the bladder urine (glass #2) be infected, the entire bacterial localization test should be repeated after the urine has been sterilized with an antibiotic. I personally prefer to use nitrofurantoin (Macrodantin) for this purpose, because this particular antibiotic is excellent for clearing up infections in the urine without being able to penetrate into the prostate and it therefore cannot interfere with the accurate determination of whether there are bacteria within the prostate gland. It is important to sterilize the bladder urine because the presence of bacteria in the bladder urine can distort the results of the bacterial localization tests. In fact, however, if the midstream urine (glass #2) is positive for infection (in the case of bladder urine a positive colony count would have more than 50,000 or 100,000 colonies of bacteria per milliliter of urine), the diagnosis of chronic bacterial prostatitis is indeed very likely. Conversely, if a patient has never had any documented infections of his bladder urine during any of the periods he has had symptoms of prostatic disease, the odds are overwhelming that he does not have and never has had chronic bacterial infection in his prostate gland. I hasten to add, at this point, that it may well turn out at some future date that bacteria or other organisms not identified at the time of this writing may ultimately turn out to be responsible for those cases of what we now call "nonbacterial prostatitis" (prostatostasis) because at the present time we are unable to find any organisms in the prostatic secretions. Whether or not many or even all of patients with nonbacterial prostatitis will ultimately be proven to indeed suffer from a bacterial or viral infection in the prostate gland is problematic, but the possibility is certainly a real one and must be considered.

At the time of the prostatic massage, if any of the prostatic fluid does travel down the urethra and outside the penis, it is obtained for culture and, of great importance, is placed on a slide for microscopic examination. When this is done and when either chronic bacterial prostatitis or chronic nonbacterial prostatitis (prostatostasis) exists, the prostatic fluid will usually have more than twenty white blood cells (pus cells) per high-power microscopic field and these will usually appear in clumps. However, as noted above, the presence of white blood cells in the prostate, which are felt to indicate inflammation in the prostate gland, have been proven to exist with remarkable frequency in large numbers of men who have had prostate biopsies for other reasons, and these are men who have no symptoms whatever referable to the prostate gland. This therefore calls into serious question whether the presence of these white blood cells (pus cells) in the prostatic secretions is related to the symptoms of which patients are complaining or is simply a red herring. Also, it should be noted that many patients with the symptoms that have been under discussion will have been found to have fewer than ten white blood cells per high-power field in their prostatic secretions; this is considered perfectly normal and not suggestive of any prostatic disease.

I do recognize that the just-described bacterial localization test involving the three glasses of urine collected along with the prostatic massage is time consuming and perhaps a bit complex and is not often used by practicing clinicians. An abbreviated form of this test has been described recently and simply calls for the culture of urine before and after the prostatic massage. If the postmassage culture is positive, the diagnosis of chronic bacterial prostatitis is suggested. Further, the absence of white blood cells in the urine prior to massage followed by the presence of white blood cells (but no bacteria) in the urine following massage is more suggestive of a chronic nonbacterial prostatitis (prostatostasis). Obviously, this simplified version of the full bacterial localization test is not nearly as complete or as accurate as the longer test, but it certainly has the advantage of being simple, and I would hope that if the full bacterial localization test is not to be carried out in a given patient, at least the pre- and postmassage test would be done before the patient is given any sort of diagnosis.

Treatment of Nonspecific Urethritis, Chronic Bacterial and Nonbacterial Prostatitis, and the Chronic Pelvic Pain Syndrome

The treatment of each of these conditions is quite different from the treatment of the other conditions; therefore it is most important that the correct diagnosis be made. Nonspecific urethritis, inflammation in the prostatic urethra, is usually treated with an antibiotic such as tetracycline or one of the synthetic tetracyclines such as doxycycline or minocycline. Chronic bacterial prostatitis, once correctly diagnosed, is usually treated with a combination of sulfa and trimethoprim (Bactrim or Septra) or with one of the fluoroquinolones such as Cipro, depending on the sensitivity to antibiotics of the specific bacterial organism found in the culture. Treatment usually continues for a minimum of three or four weeks and often for as long as two or three months. About one-third of patients, perhaps even one-half of patients, with this problem will be cured by this long-term antibiotic therapeutic regime. Sadly, many of these patients will continue to have periodic relapses of their symptoms.

Nonbacterial prostatitis (prostatostasis) is logically not treated with antibiotics although these are commonly used and it is acceptable to try antibiotic therapy for a short period of time, perhaps two weeks, on the chance that it may help. Many urologists have found that combining this with regular and frequent prostatic massage greatly helps many of these patients. Up to six weeks of such massage with a frequency of three to four times per week is carried out with the rationale of trying to "wring out," or empty as best as possible, the prostatic glands that are presumably the source of the patient's symptoms. Whether any bacteria are present in these glands is questionable, but the inflammatory cells present within the glands may be participating in the patient's discomfort and prostatic massage is done in the hope of emptying the contents of these prostatic glands. Whether such massage is preferable to frequent masturbation or intercourse which also serves to empty the prostate glands is questionable, but there are certainly those urologists who feel that the salutary effects of frequent prostatic massage are indeed better than the benefits of frequent masturbation or intercourse.

I believe that the majority of patients with the symptom complex generally associated with prostatitis do not have the prostate gland as the source of their troubles. I believe that many of these patients have symptoms that result from spasm and perhaps even from inflammation of the pelvic floor musculature, and physiotherapy to that part of the body will not uncommonly produce very happy results. Biofeedback using electromyography or pressure probes in the rectum and perineal area have helped some patients, and certainly the use of muscle relaxants such as diazepam or baclofen have helped some. Alpha blockers such as terazosin or doxazosin may also help because these can relax the musculature of the prostate and surrounding areas. There are certainly countless other therapies that have been used for this vexing condition, and for patients suffering from it, one could almost say, "If it works, use it!"

Another very simple thing that I have found to be extremely helpful in the relief of perineal pain and discomfort from this condition is to forcefully contract the muscles of the pelvis and hold the contraction just as long as you possibly can until the muscle fatigues. This would be no more than ten or twenty seconds but it should be repeated a half dozen times in a row. I have found that this often breaks up the cycle of perineal pain. The muscles that I refer to are those muscles that you squeeze when you want to shut off your urinary stream midway through the act of voiding. I think the reason this is so successful in many patients is that it tends to interrupt the spasm of the perineal muscles which I feel is often the cause of the pain associated with the chronic pelvic pain syndrome.

A word of caution before going to some of the therapies just noted, and that is that there are very definitely other organic conditions that can in some ways simulate the symptoms of chronic pelvic pain syndrome. For those patients with a urologic component to their discomfort (frequency, urgency), the possibility of interstitial cystitis must be considered and a cystoscopic exam, usually under anesthesia, is certainly indicated in these situations. Also, a urodynamic study is often of benefit in revealing a detrusor/sphincter dyssynergia which can cause some of the symptoms of the chronic pelvic pain syndrome. Finally, there can be certain conditions of the lower spine or spinal cord that can lead to similar symptoms, and often an MRI study of the lower spine is rewarding.

Unfortunately, because of the specific parts of the body that are affected, infection, inflammation, and symptoms of pain and discomfort that do seem to affect the prostate or the urethra cannot be managed in nearly as straightforward a manner as these problems could elsewhere in the body. The physician must be extremely cautious and circumspect in diagnosing and treating patients who may have one of these conditions. I have said before that there is but one giant synapse between a man's genitals and his brain, and the thought that anything could be wrong with the prostate (considered to be a genital structure) is anathema to many men and brings stark fear and severe apprehension to most others. In my experience, once a physician has told a patient that he has prostatitis, it is inevitable that the same physician will put the patient on some antibiotic. In the patient's own mind, the diagnosis of prostatitis combined with the antibiotics sends him a very strong signal that he has a bacterial infection in his prostate gland. To be sure, the physician undoubtedly really believes that a bacterial infection *does* exist despite the fact that very few physicians take the time or the trouble to do the three-glass bacterial localization test described in the previous section; they just assume the presence of a bacterial infection.

The vast majority of patients thusly diagnosed and treated with antibiotics alone will not show any improvement in their symptoms because there is no infection and no bacteria present. The net effect of the unsuccessful antibiotic therapy, however, is to worry the patient and exacerbate his concern that he is not getting any better. Most men who do not have a bacterial infection but are managed in this manner will continue to have their symptoms for a long period of time and will usually have a recurring problem of "prostatitis" for many years after the original diagnosis was made. Whenever any symptoms in the general anatomic area of the prostate occur, the patient's level of anxiety and concern will skyrocket and he will be convinced that his "infection in the prostate" has returned. Sadly, his physician will usually concur, and the cycle of inappropriate antibiotic therapy compounded by genuine anxiety begins again. Moreover, by diagnosing prostatitis and treating for an infection when none exists, the physician is putting the patient's health at risk because of the antibiotics themselves. It is not at all rare for a patient to develop an allergic manifestation to the antibiotics, and some allergic manifestations can be life threatening. It is for these reasons that the author was one of the prime movers in getting the recent National Institutes of Health Consensus Conference on Prostatitis to recommend that its name be changed to chronic pelvic pain syndrome in those cases where no bacterial infection can be found. Hopefully, this will take much of the anxiety, the fear, and the anguish from those patients suffering from this problem.

Acute Bacterial Prostatitis

Acute bacterial prostatitis is a very uncommon condition that has not been discussed before because it is *not* confused with the other prostatic problems already discussed. It results from a sudden infusion of bacteria into the prostate gland, either by direct extension from an infection in the urethra (such as nonspecific urethritis) or, very occasionally, by a blood-borne spread of bacteria from an infection somewhere else in the body. Patients with acute bacterial prostatitis are quite sick: they generally run a fever of 102 degrees or higher; have the malaise, aches, and pains that one often associates with flu; and often have low abdominal and low back pain. Since there is considerable swelling of the prostate gland caused by this infection, the inside opening of the prostatic urethra may be decreased to the point of making voiding difficult or even impossible. On such occasions, temporary catheter drainage is necessary. On digital rectal examination the prostate is acutely tender and very painful and the midstream urine specimen will invariably show 50,000 to 100,000 colonies of bacteria per milliliter of urine. If there are no bacteria in the bladder urine, the diagnosis of acute bacterial prostatitis is highly unlikely. Making the correct diagnosis of this condition in the presence of urinary infection is not at all difficult. Treatment is by antibiotics using agents such as gentamicin and Kefzol parenterally, bed rest, and careful follow-up to minimize the likelihood of resulting chronic bacterial prostatitis.

In those patients whose symptoms are thought to be from acute bacterial prostatitis but in whom the urine culture is negative and in those patients in whom acute bacterial prostatitis is *not* the diagnosis, other conditions that should be considered include appendicitis and renal colic (the passage of a kidney stone down the ureter and toward the bladder).

4

Benign
Prostatic Hyperplasia
(BPH)

A 57-year-old automobile sales agent made an appointment to see me recently. He told my nurse that it was nothing urgent, then canceled his appointment on two occasions over the next month before he finally showed up in my office. When I introduced myself, he assumed an apologetic air and told me that he had canceled the two appointments because he hated to take up my time for what he was sure did not amount to anything.

"Doc, I just don't understand it," he began. "I'm sure there is nothing wrong with me. I'm in great shape. I exercise regularly and I have never felt better." He paused and then he added, "Maybe all I need is a pill or something. I don't know, it seems to take me forever to get my water started and I guess my stream isn't very strong, either." I asked him how long he had these problems, and he said it had been about two or three years and he thought it was getting worse. He added that he had to get up two or three times during the night to go to the bathroom. "I guess what really bothers me most," he muttered, "is that when my stream finally starts, it just sort of stops pretty soon for a few seconds and starts again and then when I think I'm all done making water and I zip up my pants, more urine comes out and I wet myself."

I asked him to tell me a bit more about his delay in start-ing his urinary stream and also a bit more about just how weak his stream was.

"Well," he started, "when I feel like I've gotta go, it just seems to take forever for me to start. I guess it really isn't so long, though; maybe a half minute and even a minute. Heck," he shrugged, "it'll get better soon."

I asked him if he ever dribbled urine on the floor right around the toilet, and he suddenly looked at me and said, "How'd you know that? Yeah, that's exactly what happens and that's exactly how I know my stream isn't as good as it used to be. I have to stand right over the bowl now to keep from wet-ting the floor."

"And I'll bet that when you get an urge to make water," I said to him, "you really gotta go right away and pretty badly."

"Yep, I sure do, Doc. Is all this in my mind? I just can't imagine that anything could be wrong down there," he said, pointing to his genital area.

This patient demonstrated, with almost classic detail, the symptoms that usually accompany BPH, although many patients with this condition will not necessarily have every one of these symptoms.

Benign prostatic hyperplasia (BPH), sometimes referred to as benign prostatic hypertrophy, is a very common occur-rence and is best thought of as a natural part of aging. Quite simply, it is a process in which the prostate gland enlarges. When the condition is present, however, it does not always produce symptoms of which the patient is aware; so there may be a considerable discrepancy between the actual anatomic existence of this condition (an enlarged prostate) and the fre-quency with which it produces symptoms. An analysis of autop-sy studies reveals that over half of men who are 50 years of age or older and about three-quarters of men who are over 70 years of age actually have BPH. You should keep in mind, though, that this is an anatomic finding and reveals nothing whatever about the number of patients in whom these anatomic changes produce symptoms. A good estimate is that about one-quarter of those men who have the anatomic changes of BPH will also have symptoms that are sufficient to send them to their physician.

The cause of benign prostatic hyperplasia is poorly under-stood, although it is unquestionably related to the aging process as well as to the presence of circulating male hormones. Because of this, BPH is not found in eunuchs, for example, the very small percentage of males whose testicles were removed or became nonfunctioning prior to puberty. It is interesting to note that BPH seems in no way to be related to sexual activity, since it appears in celibate priests with the same frequency that it occurs in the general male population. It is also not apparently related in any way to sexual excesses or deprivation at any time of life. Moreover, BPH as far as we know is not related to prior infection or inflammation of the prostate or to cancer of the prostate (although prostate cancer and BPH are generally found in the same age group and can and do certainly coexist in the same individual).

The concept of BPH can be a difficult one to understand. I have found that a genuine comprehension of BPH can readily be achieved if the normal prostate gland is visualized as an apple with the core removed, as shown in Figure 1–2. The top of the apple (where the stem is) should be pictured fitting snugly against the bladder neck. The opposite end of the apple from the part with the stem may be seen to rest up against the membranous urethra, which is that part of the urethra within the sphincter muscle that a man contracts when he wants to suddenly shut off his stream while voiding (Fig. 4–1). The channel through the apple created by removing its core represents the prostatic urethra; it is through this channel that urine normally flows after leaving the bladder. This channel, the prostatic urethra, becomes obstructed when the prostate begins to enlarge, a process that usually begins around ages 40 to 45 (Fig. 4–2).

The prostatic urethra has a wall or lining just as any tubular structure in the body has a lining, and it is just beneath this lining that benign prostatic hyperplasia begins. This new growth of the prostate may occur most of the way or part of the way around the prostatic urethra. However, the prostate does not necessarily grow in a symmetrical manner. Therefore, there may be more new growth of the prostate on one side than on the other, or on the bottom (the floor) of the prostatic urethra than on either side. This new growth is made of the same types of tissue as the normal prostate gland although in different proportions. The normal prostate gland is made up of fibrous or connective tissue, muscle, and glands (see Chapter 1); the new growth of the prostate will have the same

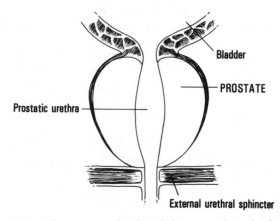

Figure 4–1   *The prostate gland and the external urethral sphincter. Note the relationship between the two. It is the external urethral sphincter that is contracted when a man wishes to shut off his urinary stream.*

Figure 4–2   *The prostate gland showing an early stage of benign prostatic hyperplasia (BPH). Note that this arises just underneath (outside) the lining of the prostatic urethra.*

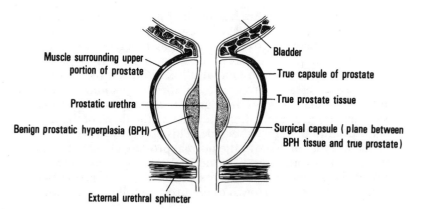

tissues but will usually have much more fibrous and muscular tissue in relation to glandular tissue.

As the growth of new prostate tissue (BPH) slowly continues, which it will usually do inexorably over a long period of time that is measured in years, it tends to grow in an outward as well as an inward direction (Fig. 4–3). When it grows toward the outside of the prostate gland, it tends to compress the true, normal prostate tissue between itself and the true capsule of the prostate gland (the skin of the apple). The point where the expanding new growth of prostate (BPH) meets the normal and true prostate tissue is called the surgical capsule. During surgery for BPH, it is only the new growth of BPH tissue that is removed (see Chapter 6). When this new BPH tissue grows toward the outside of the prostate gland, it can be felt as an enlarged prostate on digital rectal examination. However, an outward growth of the new prostate has nothing to do with bringing about any of the symptoms which a patient would notice and which are associated with BPH. Usually, though, if the new prostate tissue grows in an outward direction, it also will grow in an inward direction. This will decrease the inside size of the prostatic urethra. It is the narrowing of this channel through which the urine flows that produces the characteristic symptoms associated with benign prostatic hyperplasia (Fig. 4–4).

It is important for a patient to understand that there are only three distinct parts of the prostate gland that can cause the symptoms of BPH. These are the two lateral lobes and the middle lobe. The two lateral lobes can be felt on digital rectal examination (Fig. 4–5) and will be noted to be larger than normal if they have enlarged in an outward direction; but the middle lobe can never, under any circumstances, be felt because it is enlarging into the channel of the prostatic urethra from the floor of that urethra. This middle lobe growing up from the floor can be thought of as if the *lower* half of the apple produced a growth of BPH directly into its core while the examining finger, when placed in the rectum, is only able to feel the *upper* half of the apple. Therefore, when a rectal examination is done (Fig. 4–6) to ascertain whether the prostate is enlarged, the only parts of the prostate which can be felt and which can be causative of the symptoms of BPH are the lateral lobes. *The middle lobe, never palpable, is, however, the most common cause of the symptoms of BPH.*

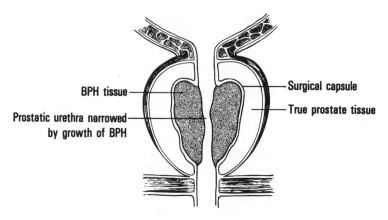

BPH tissue

Prostatic urethra narrowed
by growth of BPH

Surgical capsule

True prostate tissue

Figure 4–3   *The prostate gland showing considerable growth of benign prostatic hyperplasia (BPH). Note how it encroaches on and pushes into the channel of the prostatic urethra.*

Figure 4–4   *The prostate gland showing a severe degree of benign prostatic hyperplasia (BPH) that almost totally replaces the prostate tissue by compressing it peripherally against the true capsule of the prostate. Note particularly how the benign prostatic hyperplasia also grows in an inward direction, virtually obliterating the channel of the prostatic urethra through which urine must pass.*

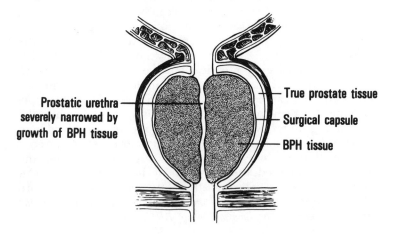

Prostatic urethra
severely narrowed by
growth of BPH tissue

True prostate tissue

Surgical capsule

BPH tissue

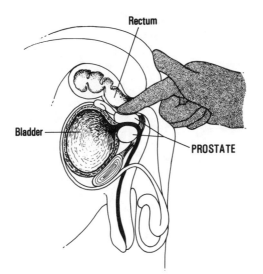

A

Figure 4–5   DIGITAL RECTAL EXAMINATION OF THE PROSTATE
GLAND
   *A. A lateral view of the examining finger palpating the prostate
gland.*
   *B. A view from straight overhead as if the patient were bent over
sharply at the waist and you were looking down from the ceiling.*

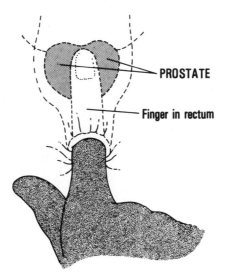

B

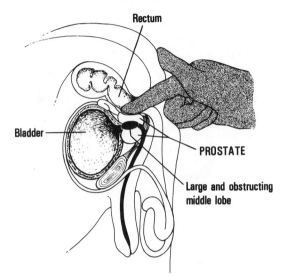

Figure 4–6   *A digital rectal examination of the prostate. Note how it is absolutely impossible for the examining finger to palpate the middle lobe of the prostate gland even though it may be severely enlarged and obstructing the flow of urine.*

Effects of BPH on the Bladder

If the process by which the new growth of prostatic tissue results in a partial or complete blockage of the channel through which the urine must flow has been understood, it is relatively easy to recognize and comprehend the symptoms that accompany this process. The act of voiding is the contraction of the bladder muscle on the one hand and the resistance to the flow of urine on the other. The channel through which the urine flows once it leaves the bladder is really just a tube that runs from the neck of the bladder all the way to the opening on the very end of the penis. Whenever anything encroaches on the interior dimensions of the tube, such as the growth of new prostate tissue, the bladder muscle has to work harder in order to carry out its mission of emptying itself during voiding. Under normal circumstances, there should be no urine left in the bladder following voiding. Bladder muscle, though perhaps more complex in its structure than most muscles in the body, will nevertheless react like any other muscle to hard work. When the bladder has to contract more forcefully in order to empty itself because of the increased resistance to the flow of urine caused by an enlarged new growth of prostate, the bladder muscle undergoes a buildup and a strengthening in much the same manner that the upper arm and chest muscles enlarge and build up when a man begins a vigorous exercise program that includes push-ups. Because of the unique nature of bladder muscle, the buildup that the bladder undergoes is an irregular one; it is not uniform throughout and generally begins in the trigone of the bladder, that part of the bladder just inside the bladder neck and on the floor of the bladder.

As the obstruction to the flow of urine becomes progressively more severe over a period of months or years (because the prostatic enlargement is usually progressive), the muscle buildup within the entire bladder, including the trigone, continues so that the bladder will have enough strength to empty itself during voiding. As long as the bladder muscle is able to build up to the point that it can overcome the resistance offered by the slowly enlarging prostate gland, it will be able to empty itself during voiding; the bladder in this condition is said to be compensated.

The new growth of BPH tissue into the channel of the prostatic urethra and the resulting obstruction to the flow of urine is usually a progressive phenomenon (although in some men it seems to progress to a certain point and then no further). The progression that usually occurs is a slow one that occurs over a period of months to years. As the obstructive process continues, the buildup of bladder muscle produces an irregular appearance known as bladder trabeculation (Fig. 4–7). Trabeculation is characterized by irregular bands of muscle that have built up within the bladder; the areas between these built-up muscle bands are recessed or "popped out" much like a Mickey Mouse balloon in which the nose and the ears pop out as you continue to blow into the balloon. These popped out areas are called cellules, and from inside the bladder they are seen as depressions in the wall of the bladder. They are not nearly as deep as the pop outs in the Mickey Mouse balloon, but they can be several millimeters and even up to a centimeter in depth. In extreme and longstand-

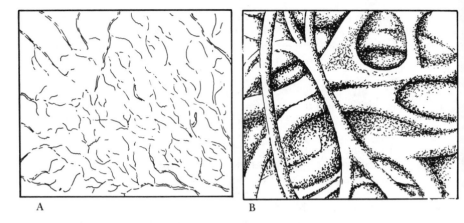

A   B

Figure 4–7   A. The interior of a normal bladder. Note the very smooth appearance of the bladder wall. The little lines indicate the normal presence of blood vessels, which are just underneath the bladder lining and are readily visible when viewed through a cystoscope.

B. The inside of the bladder showing the buildup of the bladder muscle (trabeculation). This buildup of the bladder muscle can become so severe that areas between the built-up strands of muscle actually pop out and form little outpouchings known as cellules.

C. A normal cystogram. Note the perfectly normal, smooth, and regular outline of the bladder.

D. A cystogram of a person with severe bladder outlet obstruction due to BPH. Note the marked irregularity of the bladder outline caused by the pronounced buildup of the bladder wall (trabeculation) and by the numerous outpouchings (cellules) related to this muscle buildup. The shadow in the center of the bladder is caused by a very enlarged middle lobe of the prostate gland.

C   D

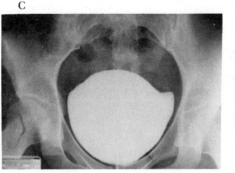
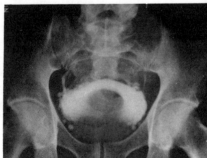

ing cases of obstruction caused by BPH, these cellules can indeed pop out for several centimeters, and they are then called diverticulae.

Symptoms of BPH

Broadly speaking there are two functions that the urinary bladder must perform: storing urine and voiding urine. When the bladder is not able to properly perform either of these functions, certain symptoms can occur (see Table 4–1).

A patient with BPH can have many, any, or even all of the symptoms that are listed under both columns "Storage" and "Voiding." Since symptoms are so subjective and hard to pin down as to severity, the American Urological Association has produced a symptom score sheet which a patient fills out and which helps the urologist to evaluate the severity of a patient's symptoms. It also is most helpful in determining symptom improvement following treatment. One of the problems in evaluating symptoms is—and this has only been realized relatively recently—that not all people with any, some, or even all of the symptoms listed in the table have benign prostatic hyperplasia. The aging bladder, in both men and women, may

Table 4–1

Symptoms of Benign Prostatic Hyperplasia or Lower Urinary Tract Symptoms (LUTS)

Storage	Voiding
Frequency	Hesitancy
Nocturia	Poor stream
Urgency	Intermittency
Bladder pain	Straining
Incontinence	Dysuria
Urge	Feeling of incomplete voiding
Stress	Postvoid micturition dribble
Continuous	

undergo changes that lead to these various symptoms in the absence of BPH. These changes, therefore, may be secondary to benign prostatic hyperplasia or they may indeed be primary bladder changes unrelated to any obstruction from the prostate.

As a general rule, patients suffering from these symptoms will indeed have them as a result of benign prostatic hyperplasia, but this is by no means always the case and it is therefore, in my opinion, necessary to determine the cause of a patient's symptoms before embarking on any invasive (surgical) form of treatment. This is particularly the case when the symptoms are predominantly those of frequency, urgency, nocturia, and incontinence since it is this group of symptoms that is more often associated with primary bladder changes that are not related to an obstructing prostate gland. The differential diagnosis between those symptoms that are caused by bladder outlet obstruction (BPH) and those symptoms caused by primary bladder changes that often accompany the aging process can most often be made by means of urodynamic studies and particularly by means of the pressure/flow study discussed in Chapter 2. This is why I feel so strongly that it is definitely preferable to have this pressure/flow study done before any invasive (surgical) treatment of what is thought to be BPH is carried out. I recognize that there is by no means uniformity of opinion among urologists on this subject, but it is one about which I feel quite strongly.

If we look at the symptoms in Table 4–1, frequency, urgency, nocturia, and incontinence are found in women as well as in men and may simply be due to an overactivity of the bladder muscle quite unrelated to any obstructed prostate gland. Similarly, the symptoms of hesitancy, weak urinary stream, straining to void, incomplete bladder emptying, and so on, can be due to poor bladder muscle contractility such as is often found in diabetic patients, patients with spinal cord damage, or patients who have had major pelvic surgery. Again, most of the time that these symptoms exist in a man over 50, it is indeed caused by bladder outlet obstruction resulting from the prostate gland. However, I believe that other factors such as those just noted can and do cause any of these symptoms and that the risk of proceeding to treating patients surgically for what is presumed to be prostatic obstruction is significant enough that I would not do it without a pressure/flow study to confirm that obstruction really is the cause of a patient's problem.

Assuming obstruction to be the cause of a patient's difficulty (as it is indeed more commonly the cause), as the process progresses it becomes more and more difficult for the patient to empty his bladder following voiding, and the resulting buildup of urine is called "residual urine." This amount may initially start out to be minimal (an ounce or two), but it is not rare to find patients with several hundred cubic centimeters or even a pint or a quart or more of urine in their bladder following voiding. This process of urine buildup following voiding is so gradual that patients are often quite unaware of their situation until they present with a complete inability to urinate, incontinence, or recurring bladder infections. The incontinence is an overflow, or a continuous loss, of urine due to the fact that the bladder is so full of residual urine there is no room for any more urine that comes down from the kidneys. It may also occur when there is a very large amount of residual urine in the bladder and bladder spasms occur. Resulting bladder infections are not uncommon when there is a pronounced inability to empty the bladder since the presence of stagnant bladder urine is a wonderful culture medium for bacteria which may be present in the urethra but which normally cause no problem as long as the bladder is emptied on a regular basis. The presence of large amounts of postvoid bladder urine with resulting infection will usually produce strongly alkaline urine with a "stablelike" odor caused by the release of ammonia resulting from the action of certain kinds of bacteria on the urine itself. This highly alkaline urine is a situation that is conducive to the formation of stones within the bladder, and these can cause considerable discomfort.

Hematuria (blood in the urine), visible to the naked eye (gross hematuria) or only when the urine is examined under a microscope (microhematuria), is a fairly common occurrence with benign prostatic hyperplasia. Indeed, BPH is one of the two most common causes of hematuria in men over 40 (bladder cancer is the other most common cause). The blood vessels supplying the urethra and bladder neck travel in the tissue just underneath its lining and this is the precise area where the BPH tissue grows. As it grows, BPH tissue stretches the blood vessels that lie on top of it; this stretching can ultimately lead to these blood vessels' bursting. If a very small blood vessel bursts, the hematuria will be seen only micro-scopically; if a larger blood vessel bursts, the hematuria will be seen with the naked eye as pink or red urine. Severe hemor-rhage from this source is a very uncommon occurrence, but it does happen and it is one indication for the surgical removal of the obstructing (and bleeding) prostatic tissue.

As the new growth of obstructing BPH tissue continues to enlarge and to produce more symptoms of increasing severi-ty, most patients eventually visit a physician to seek an under-standing and a resolution of the problem. A small and interesting minority of patients, however, are seemingly unaware of any voiding difficulties and therefore do not seek medical help. For these individuals the natural history of their disease may follow one of two routes. The first route is a pro-gression of the symptoms of obstruction until the time comes, suddenly and without warning, when the patient has the severe discomfort of acute urinary retention and is unable to pass any urine at all. Prompt treatment of this condition requires the passage of a catheter into the bladder in order to drain the urine. Some patients are then seemingly without any particular symptoms for an indefinite period of time following this one-time catheterization, and nothing definitive is usually done for these patients. However, other patients having an episode of acute urinary retention have repeated such episodes and these people inevitably require surgical relief from their disease.

The second and far more serious route that BPH may very infrequently follow is that of progressive back pressure on the kidneys, uremic poisoning, and even death. Once the bladder has become decompensated, the residual urine which remains after voiding invariably increases to larger and larger quantities; in this small group of patients, the drainage of urine from the kidneys is blocked because the large amount of urine already in the bladder prevents any more urine from entering. The high pressure in the bladder resulting from the great quantity of urine in it is transmitted back up to the kid-neys where normal kidney function, which is to filter blood and thereby remove various waste products, is severely impaired. Uremic poisoning, which results when these waste products are not filtered and removed from the kidneys, sets in and can be diagnosed by measuring the blood levels of cre-atinine and urea nitrogen, two of the waste products that must be removed (see Chapter 2). If satisfactory drainage of the bladder (and therefore of the kidneys) is not brought about promptly, coma and death may ensue.

A most interesting question that is usually asked is: Why and how is it possible for an individual who has BPH that is severe enough to lead to acute urinary retention or even death not to be aware of the symptoms of BPH at a much earlier stage that would have led him to a physician for help? I feel that there are three possible explanations for this seemingly extraordinary, albeit very uncommon fact. First, the symptoms of bladder outlet obstruction (BPH) can be subtle in their onset and are usually very slow in their progression. It is therefore certainly a possibility that a patient can grow so accustomed to his symptoms of bladder outlet obstruction that he cannot remember when he did *not* have them. Thus he considers the symptoms to be normal for him, thereby not requiring a visit to his physician.

Second, since many men regard the prostate as a genital structure, and nothing is more important to them than their genitals—perhaps even life itself—these men are subconsciously unwilling to admit that they have any symptoms of prostatic disease and so completely deny all symptoms associated with the prostate gland. Whether this is done consciously or unconsciously, the result is that the patient does deny all symptoms associated with the prostate gland. The patient cited at the beginning of this chapter, for example, certainly had a problem with disease denial, although not to the degree where he failed to seek help.

Third, and a real consideration for many who have limited financial means and have not been brought up in the mainstream of society, is that every entry into the health care system is a foreboding process, a costly one, and one that is to be avoided if at all possible. For these individuals the symptoms of bladder outlet obstruction often represent nothing more than additional problems to the many already present in their troubled lives and just are not severe enough to warrant a visit to a physician.

Overall, I estimate that the vast majority of patients ultimately seeking treatment for the symptoms of BPH do indeed come to the physician because of one or more of the symptoms already noted. A small percentage of patients, well under 5 percent of those with BPH, will present themselves initially to a physician or to an emergency room with either the problem of an inability to void (acute urinary retention) or the problems associated with uremic poisoning, which generally are severe weakness and fatigue.

It is worth mentioning once again that the diverse set of symptoms that have been under discussion as associated with benign prostatic hyperplasia (BPH) may occasionally not be related in any way to BPH. They may rather be related to primary bladder problems such as might result from diabetes wherein the bladder is unable to empty itself or from changes the bladder undergoes associated with aging that lead to urgency, frequency, nocturia, and even urge incontinence. In both of these examples, the bladder symptoms present are not caused by BPH but are primary to the bladder.

Physical Examination

Your doctor will very probably begin by feeling your lower abdomen in order to detect whether your bladder is full. This is done simply because one of the eventual occurrences with BPH may be a significant residual urine which may be large enough in amount to be detected because of distention of the urinary bladder. In very unusual circumstances, a full bladder may reach all the way to the umbilicus, but it is not uncommon to find a bladder that is enlarged to the point halfway between the pubic hair and the umbilicus. This will happen with a patient who is not able to empty his bladder on voiding and carries about a pint of residual urine after voiding.

Digital rectal examination of the prostate gland is the only other part of the physical examination that is germane to the diagnosis of BPH, although it must again be emphasized that it is certainly *not* a definitive examination since it cannot unequivocally determine if the patient does or does not have clinically significant BPH. Even more importantly, it cannot reveal whether any BPH that *may* be present is actually producing obstruction to the flow or urine. This is because, as we have seen, it is often the middle lobe of the prostate gland that is most likely to produce symptoms of bladder outlet obstruction, and the middle lobe is *never* palpable on rectal examination. The lateral lobes of the prostate gland, on the other hand, are readily palpable on digital rectal examination, but enlargement of these lobes is only suggestive and certainly not diagnostic of obstruction to the flow of urine. As a general rule, if the lateral lobes are enlarged in an outward direction so that they feel enlarged to the examiner's finger, the chances are good that these same lateral lobes will also be enlarged in an inward direction and will encroach on the channel of the prostatic urethra and may then produce symptoms of obstruction to the flow of urine. An equally general rule is that if the lateral lobes are not palpably enlarged on digital rectal examination, they probably are not enlarged in an inward direction either.

It should be clear, therefore, that the prostate gland that is only minimally enlarged or not enlarged at all tells the examining physician absolutely nothing about whether there is any middle lobe enlargement that could be quite significant; further, enlargement of the lateral lobes is suggestive but by no means conclusive that lateral lobe obstruction to the flow of urine exists; finally, lateral lobes that are not enlarged on digital rectal examination suggest the absence of any lateral lobe obstruction to the flow of urine. In addition to the two lateral lobes, the posterior lobe is the only other lobe of the prostate that is palpable on rectal examination, and this lobe is never a participant in the process of BPH.

In fact, the most important information to be gained from the digital rectal examination is probably whether the patient's prostate gland is suggestive of malignancy or is probably benign. A second bit of information to be gained from the rectal examination is an estimate of how large the prostate gland may be so as to give the urologist an early signal as to the optimum surgical approach (if surgery is contemplated).

Diagnostic Studies for Symptomatic Benign Prostatic Hyperplasia

Urine Analysis and Urine Culture

The urine analysis is a standard part of the examination of any patient known or thought to have BPH. Even though this test does not directly contribute to the diagnosis of this condition, it is important for the physician to know if the patient has more than a very few white blood cells (pus cells) in the urine since this would suggest, but certainly not prove, the possibility of a urinary tract infection. Also, it is important to know if there are any red blood cells in the urine (microhematuria) since the presence of blood in the urine pretty well mandates that kidney x-rays (an excretory urogram) be obtained prior to any possible prostate surgery. Although red blood cells are a common finding with BPH, they also can be a warning of serious disease in the kidneys or bladder which could be detected by the excretory urogram. Examination of the urine can reveal other important things about the general state of a patient's health such as the presence of sugar or protein in the urine (both abnormal).

A urine culture may be indicated if white blood cells are present in the urine. This urine culture can document with certainty the presence or absence of an infection. Should one be present, it must be treated promptly. Infection, particularly repeated infections in the bladder, provide a strong indication for considering prostate surgery in a patient. It is presumed that the recurrent infections are due to an inability to empty the bladder following voiding.

Blood Studies

There are no available blood studies that will diagnose benign prostatic hyperplasia; however, several blood studies are generally carried out during the course of a patient's evaluation for BPH and are virtually always done prior to any contemplated prostate surgery. One of these is the determination of the blood creatinine level, since this is one of the best and certainly the simplest method of evaluating how well a patient's kidneys are functioning. An abnormal elevation of the creatinine level may be important for two reasons: first, it may represent a valid reason all by itself to consider prostate surgery in order to restore normal kidney function; second, any contemplated prostate surgery is best deferred until kidney function has been improved to its optimum, usually by means of prolonged catheterization. It is not at all unusual in some patients with BPH to find a large amount of residual urine that has been present for a prolonged period of time and has resulted in an elevation of the blood creatinine level. This usually means that a person has already suffered renal damage from back pressure on the kidneys. Such an elevation of the creatinine level does not necessarily mean that a patient is too sick for surgery, but it does mean that surgery should ideally be deferred until the kidney function is improved.

The other blood study that is sometimes done when a patient is being evaluated for BPH is the prostate specific antigen (PSA) level. Mild elevation of the prostate specific antigen (PSA) may be seen with BPH, particularly when the prostate is quite large. However, it usually requires further evaluation to be certain that prostate cancer is not present (see Chapter 2). High levels of PSA may well indicate the presence of prostate cancer although the reader should note that having an infection in the bladder or in the prostate can lead to a spurious elevation of the PSA level. Generally speaking, neither of these findings (an elevated creatinine level or an elevated PSA level) would alter the requirements of treating a patient's symptoms of bladder outlet obstruction. However, it might delay such treatment while the patient is placed on catheter drainage in the hope of lowering the blood creatinine level, or it may well modify the surgical approach or even the timing of the surgery if it is felt that prostatic carcinoma exists (see Chapter 6).

X-ray and Other Imaging Studies

Many urologists like to visualize the entire urinary tract prior to any contemplated prostate surgery and for this reason an excretory urogram has traditionally been done prior to prostate surgery. If affords an opportunity to visualize and evaluate both the upper (kidneys and ureters) and lower (bladder and urethra) urinary tract. The excretory urogram can assure me that my patient's kidneys are perfectly normal in appearance without any stones, tumors, obstructions, or other abnormalities that are best discovered before surgery. Similarly, the lower urinary tract can also be evaluated for bladder stones which may result from bladder infections caused by BPH, and finally, the excretory urogram is useful for estimating the size of the prostate enlargement (Fig. 4–8).

The trend nowadays, however, is not to do an excretory urogram prior to surgery but to study the kidneys by means of ultrasound (Fig. 4–9) or a kidney scan (Fig. 4–10). Both of these studies can pretty well assure the absence of any signifi-

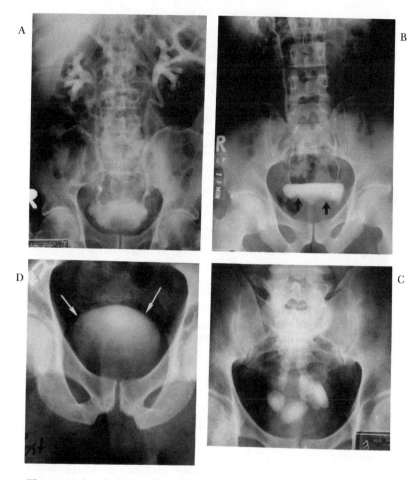

Figure 4–8   EXCRETORY UROGRAMS *(from different patients)*
demonstrating some of the abnormalities associated with benign pros-
tatic hyperplasia (BPH). Compare these with a normal excretory uro-
gram in Figure 2–1.

A. *Obstructed upper urinary tract (kidneys and ureters) caused*
by BPH.

B. *A marked elevation of the base of the bladder (arrows) caused*
by enlarged lateral lobes of the prostate (BPH).

C. *Multiple stones within the bladder caused by high residual*
urine with resulting infection in the bladder. This film is taken prior
to injection of any contrast material.

D. *High residual urine seen on the postvoiding film. The inabil-*
ity to empty the bladder is caused by the large and obstructing
prostate. The arrows indicate the outline of the enlarged bladder,
which is filled with contrast medium.

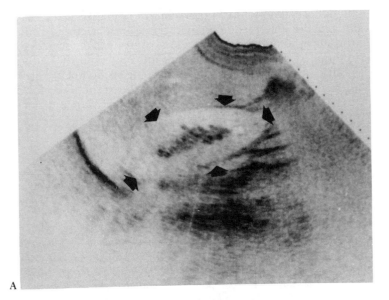

A

Figure 4–9 ULTRASOUND OF THE KIDNEYS

 A. A perfectly normal kidney identified by the arrows.

 B. An obstructed kidney with dilation of the collecting system of the kidney caused by an enlarged prostate with back pressure on the kidney. Arrows identify the dilated collecting system of the kidney.

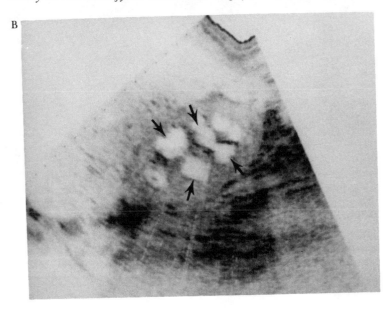

B

cant abnormalties in the kidneys, but I emphasize again that if any gross or microscopic hematuria is present, an excretory urogram is far and away the preferable study to determine the presence or absence of any significant lesions in the kidney. Because of fiscal awareness, many urologists do not carry out any evaluation of the upper urinary tract (except on occasions where there has been micro- or gross hematuria), and this is certainly perfectly acceptable.

Figure 4–10   ABNORMAL RENAL SCAN
   Marked obstruction and enlargement of the kidney on the left caused by an enlarged and obstructing prostate gland. On the photograph on the left, note that the left kidney remains very dense over a progressive time interval as the injected radioisotope remains in the kidney and cannot drain out because of the obstruction. In the photograph on the right, an injection of a diuretic (a substance that makes the kidneys produce more urine) has been given to the patient, and this serves to exaggerate even more the blockage to the left kidney. Note also the obstruction and dilation of the left ureter (the tube that drains the kidney). For comparison with a normal renal scan, see Figure 2–2.

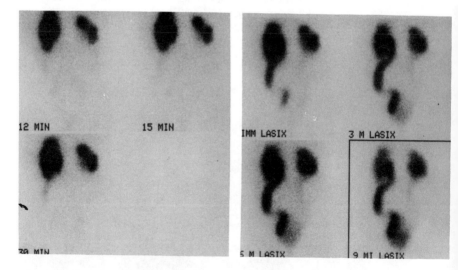

Urodynamic Studies

As noted in Chapter 2, these studies provide a reasonably accurate and very reproducible means of determining quantitatively how well the bladder is carrying out its two functions of storage of urine and voiding of urine. I cannot emphasize enough that the symptoms associated with BPH can infrequently be caused by primary bladder problems and not bladder problems that are secondary to the obstructing prostate gland. This very important differentiation, if made before any contemplated surgical treatment, can go far toward minimizing those postoperative results where the patient is not improved or, even more upsetting, the patient is worse than he was before the surgery. A pressure/flow study such as was described in Chapter 2 is carried out, and the bladder pressure is monitored as the bladder is slowly filled and then at the time that voiding begins. This voiding is done around a small catheter that has been used to fill the bladder, and the rate of flow in milliliters per second of the urine coming out around the catheter is measured also.

Ideally, the pressure within a patient's bladder as it is being filled should remain very low and quite constant until the bladder is at its capacity. At that point, the patient voids, and a normal voiding pressure is 30 or 40 centimeters of water with a normal flow rate of something over 15 millileters per second. If the bladder pressure at the time of voiding is as high as 50–60 centimeters of water while the urine flow rate during voiding is less than 10 millileters per second, a diagnosis of bladder outlet obstruction may safely be made. Also, if the pressure within the bladder at the time of voiding is 100 centimeters of water or higher, regardless of the flow rate when urine is voided, a diagnosis of bladder outlet obstruction may also be made. A very important caveat is that these elevated bladder pressures just noted must be recorded when the patient is told to void at the time that he feels his bladder is full and the patient must not use any of his voluntary abdominal muscles to help expel the urine. The latter gives a spurious elevation of the bladder pressure which does not bear any particular relationship to obstruction that may be present or absent.

Also, when the bladder is filling, some bladders will show involuntary "spikes" of increased pressure which are abnormal since the pressure within the bladder should normally remain fairly constant and flat until the bladder capacity has been reached. These involuntary spikes of pressure within the bladder, even though they may be 100 centimeters of water or higher, are indicative not of bladder outlet obstruction but merely of involuntary bladder contraction. It is these contractions that help to diagnose an overactive bladder, and whether this is a primary bladder problem or secondary to bladder outlet obstruction is dependent on the bladder pressure and urine flow rate at the time of voiding.

In addition, the material that is used to fill the bladder is frequently radio opaque so that as the bladder is filled and particularly during voiding, fluoroscopy may be carried out, and this can sometimes specifically identify the location of the bladder outlet obstruction. Usually, however, this fluoroscopic portion of the procedure is not necessary although it is always of interest to document fluoroscopically exactly where the obstructing area may be, recognizing that it is almost always at the bladder neck or within the prostatic urethra.

As I noted in Chapter 2, these urodynamic studies are by no means carried out by most urologists prior to any contemplated prostate surgical procedure. I do feel strongly, however, that they are very valuable in trying to predict with the greatest possible degree of accuracy which patients can be expected to have a salutary result from prostate surgery and to avoid surgery in those patients who have not been urodynamically demonstrated to be obstructed.

Cystoscopic Examination

The diagnosis of bladder outlet obstruction caused by benign prostatic hyperplasia can often be made after a careful history is obtained from a patient; the history will invariably disclose many of the symptoms already noted. Physical examination is of minimal help in making or confirming the diagnosis even if a patient happens to have a palpably enlarged bladder with a large amount of residual urine in it. Although the odds are that this would be produced by bladder outlet obstruction caused by the prostate gland, there is always the possibility that the large amount of residual urine is caused by a primary bladder problem such as diabetes could produce. The digital rectal examination of the prostate gland is always done and may at times be helpful if the lateral lobes are consistently enlarged to palpation. However, it is certainly not a major determinant in the ultimate diagnosis of bladder outlet obstruction due to BPH. The blood and urine tests certainly cannot diagnose BPH, and even the excretory urogram can only strongly suggest the existence of this condition by demonstrating a large amount of residual urine in the bladder or a negative shadow in the bladder portion of the x-ray caused by enlarged lobes of the prostate (see Fig. 4–8). The pressure/flow study, if it has been done, is without question, in my opinion, the definitive way of diagnosing bladder outlet obstruction. By combining all of the various studies just noted, the physician can be quite comfortable with the diagnosis of BPH without the need to perform a cystoscopic examination.

Nevertheless, cystoscopy is indeed often carried out and there are two principal reasons for this: first, to estimate as best as possible the size of the prostate gland so as to plan the optimum surgical approach (see Chapter 6) and, second, to evaluate the bladder itself to be sure there is no coexisting pathology such as a bladder tumor. Most often, this cystoscopic examination can be carried out at the same time as the planned surgical procedure if indeed a surgical procedure is contemplated. The reader should bear in mind, however, that cystoscopy *cannot* assess the degree of *functional* obstruction; that is, cystoscopy cannot by itself tell a urologist whether a given patient requires surgery for BPH. Some urologists prefer to do the cystoscopic examination in the office prior to any contemplated surgery, while other urologists may choose to do the cystoscopy in the operating room at the time of the planned surgical procedure.

Indications for Treatment of BPH

Subjective Indications

The indications for the treatment of bladder outlet obstruction caused by BPH can perhaps best be placed into two broad groups of conditions which I like to consider *subjective* and *objective*. This applies to any of the therapeutic modalities that urologists may employ to treat BPH and it includes watchful waiting when this is appropriate, pharmacologic treatment (using various drugs to help the patient urinate better), so-called minimally invasive procedures which are still classified as surgical procedures, and "true" surgical procedures which are those which have been proven to be beneficial over a long period of time.

The first broad indication for treatment of BPH should be considered under the heading of *subjective indications*. These are the complaints and the symptoms as stated by the patient; they are said to be subjective because it is difficult for a physician to measure them in a quantitative manner. Symptoms are subjective because the causative stimuli produce differing symptoms (or no symptoms at all) in different individuals. For example, when a patient says that he has a "weak urinary stream" or "trouble starting his stream," it must be obvious that what one person would call a weak urinary stream would not necessarily be so to another. The perception of stimuli, therefore, will vary from person to person as will even the reporting of identical symptoms. The difference between the stoic individual and the hypochondriac is considerable, and while the vast majority of people are at neither of these extremes, the great middle ground between them still leaves much room for differing reports.

For these reasons, I rarely tell a patient that treatment is indicated on the basis of his symptoms alone. I much prefer to wait until the patient himself requests that something be done to relieve him of his symptoms. In my experience, patients who announce that they are ready for treatment invariably do better than those who are told that they should have treatment, and this is particularly true if treatment is to be surgical. To sum up, for those patients in whom relief of symptoms is the *only* indication for treatment, I believe that watchful waiting is the best course to follow. This means that I watch the patient to make sure his renal function does not deteriorate and I wait for him to tell me if and when he wants specific treatment for the symptoms. In other words, in patients having only the *subjective* indications for treatment, it is my general practice to let the patient make his own decision as to whether these symptoms should be treated.

Objective Indications for Treatment

These are the indications that are measurable and are not dependent on a patient's interpretation. Moreover, they are reasonably precise and specific enough that several physicians seeing the same patient will agree on the findings. A high postvoid residual urine, for example, is something that can be accurately measured (in milliliters). A heavily trabeculated bladder is something that can be observed through a cystoscope or seen when an excretory urogram is performed. Recurrent bladder infections can be documented by bacterial cultures of the patient's urine. Acute urinary retention or overflow incontinence are findings that can be agreed on by anyone witnessing them. Back pressure on the ureters and kidneys as seen on an excretory urogram or on ultrasound are also examples of objective findings as would be a rise in blood creatinine level which is usually an accompaniment of back pressure on the kidneys. Any one of these findings would indicate to me the need for treatment of the patient's bladder outlet obstruction. More than one finding indicates a more urgent need for treatment. Yet another objective indication for treatment which does not occur very often is bleeding from spontaneous rupture of the blood vessels in the prostatic urethra that have been stretched to the point of spontaneous bursting by the new growth of prostate. Usually, such bleeding stops spontaneously, but it not infrequently recurs.

To sum up, then, the objective indications for treatment include residual urine (generally over 100–150 millileters), recurrent bladder infection, bladder stones, decreasing kidney function (rising blood creatinine levels), obstruction to the drainage of the kidneys, acute urinary retention, and overflow incontinence.

A word about residual urine. The larger the volume of residual urine, the greater the need for treatment. Since residual urine is usually a late finding in the ongoing growth process of benign prostatic hyperplasia, it is specious to think that treatment should not be contemplated until a large residual urine is present. On the other hand when it is present, treatment is probably mandatory, and the larger the volume of residual urine, the greater the need for treatment.

Pharmacologic Treatment

When the patient's indications for treatment all fall in the *subjective* category and the patient wants relief of his symptoms, I will invariably start by recommending pharmacologic rather than surgical (interventional) treatment. When the patient's signs of bladder outlet obstruction fall into the *objective* category, pharmacologic treatment is certainly worth a therapeutic try and I will usually give it a try if the patient desires this. But in my experience pharmacologic treatment is best suited for patients having *only* the subjective findings associated with bladder outlet obstruction. For patients having the objective signs of bladder outlet obstruction, there is generally a need for more definitive therapy, either minimally invasive or "true" surgical treatment.

The pharmacologic treatment of benign prostatic hyperplasia involves two broad categories of medication although there are many, many others that are in various stages of investigation and may ultimately be proven to be as good as, or better than, the medications currently being used.

The first group of drugs are called alpha blockers, and these work directly on the smooth muscles of the bladder neck and the prostate gland itself to relax these muscles thereby enlarging somewhat the channel in the prostate urethra through which the urine flows. These alpha blockers work on the fibromuscular portion of the prostate gland and lead to a significant decrease in symptoms (subjective) in many patients; they also lead to an improvement in urine flow rate as measured in cubic centimeters per second (which is an objective measurement) in many patients. In evaluating the merit of drugs used to treat benign prostatic hyperplasia, it is really most important to seek some objective parameter to evaluate the efficacy of the drug being used.

Although it is the subjective aspect (the symptoms) of voiding difficulties that most concern the patient and although we are in fact interested in relieving the patient's symptoms, it nevertheless is a fact that patients given placebos will often say that their symptoms are improved. That is because they so desperately want this to be the case that they perceive it to be. Remember, as noted earlier in this book, most men believe the prostate is a genital structure and are frankly loath to admit or recognize that anything could be wrong with any part of their genital apparatus. They therefore are fairly grasping at straws when given any sort of drug; they want desperately for that drug to work. I suppose that as long as a patient says he is better that is the major point of treatment, but it must be realized that for proper evaluation of any medication's efficacy, there has to be some objective means (such as a flow rate) of finding exactly what it is doing. It is for this reason that the medical literature is just as interested in improvement of urinary flow rate as it is in symptom improvement when new drugs are introduced and used.

In any case, alpha blockers do indeed improve the symptoms of many patients both subjectively and objectively, and probably 50 to 60 percent of people on these drugs would say that they void more satisfactorily as a result of the drug's use. A somewhat lower percentage of patients will have an objective improvement in voiding flow rate, but still, probably more than half of the patients taking these drugs report that they are happy with them. The alpha blockers that are most in use are terazosin (Hytrin) and doxazosin (Cardura). Both of these drugs were originally developed to treat high blood pressure, and most patients on these drugs do experience a small drop in blood pressure that is somewhere between 5 and 10 millimeters systolic but about 5 percent of these patients have a large enough drop in blood pressure that they report feeling lightheaded or dizzy. A very small percentage of these patients report other side effects such as ankle swelling. Therefore, some of these patients will discontinue use of the drug and other therapeutic means must then be employed. A newer drug called tamsulosin (Flomax) has the same salutary effects on the prostate and bladder neck as terazosin and doxazosin, but it is more specific for this area and has less of a likelihood of affecting the blood pressure. Therefore, it is a drug that may well be used in patients on various other blood pressure medications without any concern about lowering the blood pressure too much. Tamsulosin, therefore, is a good drug to use in patients who cannot tolerate either terazosin or doxazosin.

The second broad type of drug used to treat benign prostatic hyperplasia is a drug that acts at the cellular level in the prostate gland by blocking the conversion of testosterone to dihydrotestosterone, and it is this latter substance that is most responsible for the growth of the prostate gland and the maintenance of its size. This drug has the generic name of finasteride and the trade name of Proscar, and it exerts its effects on the glandular elements within the prostate gland. It must be borne in mind, however, that the fibromuscular portion of BPH is much larger than the glandular portion in a ratio of roughly five to one, and so it is not surprising that the alpha blockers, generally speaking, work for many more people than finasteride. Finasteride is particularly suited, however, to those patients having a large prostate gland, and this means a prostate that is larger than 40 or 50 grams, a size that probably is only present in about 20 percent of patients who have BPH. It should also be noted that Proscar generally takes up to six months or even longer to achieve its maximum benefit, and while it does serve to shrink the prostate gland by as much as 20 to 30 percent of its original volume, it is only beneficial in patients who have a large prostate to start with. A small percentage of men, perhaps 3 to 4 percent, will experience sexual side effects from the finasteride such as decreased libido, decreased erectile ability, or ejaculatory problems, but about half of the people having these problems will find that the problems resolve after they have been on the drug for about a year. It should be borne in mind that both the alpha blocker and the finasteride must be taken indefinitely if their beneficial effects are to be maintained. Stopping taking either of these drugs would result in the patient's voiding problems returning to their level before therapy was started.

To sum up pharmacologic treatment, I believe that for those patients who have only the *subjective* symptoms of bladder outlet obstruction and who want to receive treatment, pharmacologic treatment is indeed the optimum way to begin. I generally start with an alpha blocker because if it is going to help the patient, salutory results will be seen in two to three weeks and because I believe it has a much greater likelihood of helping the patient than finasteride. On the other hand, patients with a very large prostate may indeed be helped significantly by finasteride, and I will use that drug in such patients. While I see nothing wrong with starting pharmacologic treatment in patients having the *objective* signs of bladder outlet obstruction, specifically high postvoid residual urine, recurrent infections, acute urinary retention, back pressure on the kidneys, and so on, in my experience pharmacologic therapy does not usually serve to eliminate these findings and one of the surgical interventions is usually required.

Finally, a word about the pressure/flow studies about which I have said so much while emphasizing how important I believe them to be. I do not feel it at all necessary to do pressure/flow studies prior to starting a patient on pharmacotherapy because there is very little lost by instituting this therapy even if it does not work. On the other hand, before I would recommend to a patient any of the surgical interventions, whether one of the minimally-invasive or one of the "true" surgical interventions, I would certainly do a pressure/flow study because I feel that this greatly increases the likelihood of such intervention being successful.

Alternative Medical Treatments

In the course of my practice I have found many patients who tell me that they are using one sort of herbal remedy or another, usually recommended by friends, a men's magazine, or a pharmacist. My feeling about this is that if the patient feels he is being helped by this over-the-counter medication, then that is fine, and I encourage him to continue with it assuming that he has only the subjective indications for treatment. As long as a patient does not have any of the objective indications for treatment such as decreasing kidney function, recurring infections, a high postvoid residual urine, and so on, I am perfectly happy to let my patient decide whether a medicine that he is taking makes him feel better and void more efficaciously. There is no question in my mind that such herbal remedies rarely improve the voiding flow rate and could not therefore pass many scientific tests of validity as far as objectively improving a patient with bladder outlet obstruction. However, I do not think this is important as long as the patient feels he is better and he is happy. One such herbal remedy is saw palmetto, and many of my patients swear by it. When my patients are happy with this or any other herbal or over-the-counter medication, I never pooh-pooh it and I am encouraging to my patients in their efforts to treat themselves. I do not believe for one minute that we physicians have all the answers in the world, and where the patient responds well to a therapy, whether something I am giving him or something he has found for himself, I encourage it and I accept it.

Watchful Waiting

This was alluded to earlier as one of the forms of treatment for bladder outlet obstruction caused by BPH. I do indeed consider this a form of treatment because it by no means implies ignoring the patient. Rather, for those patients who have only the *subjective* symptoms of bladder outlet obstruction and who are not bothered by those symptoms to the point that they want treatment, I truly believe that a course of watchful waiting is a wise and prudent course to follow. This means that the patient should be seen at intervals that do not exceed once a year and may even be more frequent than this. At such intervals the patient is again asked about his symptoms and whether he wants any treatment for them, his urine is again examined to be sure there is no infection in it (such infections are not always symptomatic), and a blood creatinine level is again done to be sure there has been no decrease in kidney function caused by possible back pressure on the kidney. Finally, an ultrasound examination of the bladder to determine the postvoid residual urine (if any) is also ideally done again. In this manner, the patient is indeed being treated, and this course of watchful waiting can continue indefinitely until either the patient determines that he wants a more active form of treatment or there is objective evidence that he requires such active treatment.

5

Cancer of
the Prostate

I saw two patients recently whom I would like to tell you about. The first of these patients was fortunate; the second was not. A 56-year-old Mercedes-Benz mechanic was referred to me by one of the best family medicine practitioners in my area because of an elevation in his PSA level. The patient told me that he had gone to his family doctor for a routine physical exam and been told that although the digital rectal examination of his prostate felt perfectly normal, his PSA level was reported as 5.1, somewhat above the generally accepted level of PSA for his age (see Chapter 2). He went on to say that his doctor had referred him to me for my opinion about what to do next.

"Honest, doctor, I don't see what the fuss is about," the patient said to me. "I don't have any pain, I pass my water like I did twenty years ago, and nothing hurts me."

I did a rectal examination and I felt this man's prostate and told him that although there were no abnormalities on the rectal examination, I remained concerned about the elevation in his PSA level. I recommended to this gentleman that he have an ultrasound-guided prostate biopsy (see Chapter 2), and he agreed to this. The biopsies showed that this man did indeed have cancer of the prostate. Why did I say earlier that this man was fortunate even though he was found to have cancer? I said it because he had his cancer discovered before it had spread and surgical removal of the entire prostate will hopefully cure this man. He was indeed fortunate to have had a family physician who performed annual digital rectal examinations of the prostate and ordered annual PSA blood tests and who then promptly referred for consultation any findings that did not seem normal.

The second patient was a 58-year-old sales agent who called my office for an appointment because of a backache. He told my nurse that he thought he must have kidney trouble and therefore he thought he should see a urologist.

As soon as he walked into my office, he pointed to the middle of his low back and told me, "Doc, the pain in there is really getting to me! I have had it for about a month now, it's not getting any better, and there doesn't seem to be anything I can do to relieve it." He went on to say he had assumed it was a kidney infection because his wife had once been told she had a kidney infection when she had similar pain. This gentleman also told me that he did have a family physician whom he would see whenever he felt sick but the last time he had seen that physician was about a year ago. He told me that the family physician never did a digital rectal examination and never ordered any PSA blood tests because he didn't believe there was much benefit to those tests.

When I did a rectal examination of his prostate gland, I was not at all surprised to find that a good part of that gland was rock hard and strongly suggestive of cancer. Subsequent x-rays of his back confirmed my suspicion that his back pain was caused by the spread of his prostate cancer to the bones of his lower spine and pelvis. The prostate was biopsied to prove the diagnosis of cancer and palliative treatment was recommended. This type of treatment, by definition, means that the patient's cancer has progressed beyond the point where cure can be anticipated and therefore it is simply palliative. Treatment is directed at making a patient as comfortable as possible and prolonging life as long as it still has a degree of quality.

Unhappily, this patient's story is not rare. Even in this day when the PSA blood test is able to detect prostate cancers at a very early and potentially curative stage, there are many primary care physicians who do not believe in the value of this blood test, and therefore patients like the one just noted do still present from time to time with what is obviously advanced and incurable prostate cancer.

Incidence of Prostate Cancer

Prostate cancer is a very common form of cancer and, if skin cancers are excluded, the most frequent form of malignancy occurring in men, accounting for about 180,000 new cases in 1999. Looking at the statistics from another point of view, almost 30 percent of all nonskin cancers diagnosed in men are of prostatic origin. Overall, prostatic cancer is the second most common cause of cancer death in men after lung cancer, and about 37,000 men died of this condition in 1999. The obvious discrepancy between the incidence of prostate cancer and the death rate of this cancer is a clear reflection of the fact that in many cases prostatic cancer is of very low-grade malignancy and men die *with* it rather than *from* it. It has been estimated that about one-third of men in the United States over 50 years of age may have cancer of the prostate gland, and yet only a small fraction of these men will succumb to this disease.

The actual size, in cubic centimeters, of the prostate cancer in any given man, as well as the microscopic appearance of the tumor—whether it is a low-grade or high-grade malignancy—are the determinants of whether the carcinoma will act in a relatively benign way by spreading very slowly over many years or in a more malignant fashion with more rapid spread through the body over a period of relatively few years. Prostatic cancer is uncommon in men under 50, but from then on it manifests itself with increasing frequency, reaching a peak in the over-75 age group when as many as 60 to 75 percent of all men may have this condition in one form or another, but usually in the relatively milder form of low-grade malignancy. Though many hypotheses and interesting observations have been made, the cause of prostate cancer remains unknown.

There has recently been much written in the lay and the medical presses about the idea that many men with prostate cancer that is localized to the prostate gland do not need to have any treatment other than watchful waiting with regular examination, including periodic PSA levels which may be of help in determining if the cancer is growing. This publicity has come about because of the known fact that the great majority of men with prostate cancer do indeed die *with* it and not *from* it. Statistically, if great numbers of prostate cancer patients are included in a study, it is safe to say that prostate cancer will not be the cause of death for the majority of these patients. However, for any one given patient this just cannot be said. Cancer, by definition, grows, spreads, and kills. The questions for any specific patient are what is that patient's life expectancy absent the prostate cancer and can it therefore be safely predicted that the patient would die from some other cause before the prostate cancer could cause his death? Obviously, the answers to these questions are impossible to predict, but there are certain factors that can help with these predictions.

The most important is probably the patient's age at the time of diagnosis, and the younger the patient is, the more obvious is the need for definitive treatment of the cancer and not a course of watchful waiting. What age am I referring to when I say this? I believe that any patient under age 70 should certainly be encouraged to have either surgical or radiation treatment for his prostate cancer. Over age 70 the answer to this question is not quite as clear and one can certainly make a cogent argument for watchful waiting. The age at which a patient's father died and the cause of death can sometimes be a tip-off about a patient's genetic determinants of life expectancy, particularly if there is a strong family history, for example, of cardiac disease and death by the early seventies or before. My general rule of thumb is that if a patient has ten years or fewer of life expectancy, I recommend a course of watchful waiting. I do, however, always encourage my patients to express their preference, and if they prefer to be treated, regardless of age, I will certainly go along with them as far as referring them for radiation therapy. I do not, as a general rule, recommend or perform surgery on a patient who is much past 70 years of age.

Finally, a note about watchful waiting. This definitely does not mean benign neglect but rather following the patient annually or semiannually with PSA blood tests with the anticipation that eventually the cancer will have spread to the extent that it becomes objectively symptomatic (often with bone pain), and at that point I recommend hormone therapy to the patient as a palliative measure. This hormone therapy is described later in this chapter and the optimum starting time for such hormone therapy can be variable. Certainly it should be started by the time that cancer has spread to other parts of the body, but for many patients it is started considerably before this time, often at the patient's request. However, although it is quite certain that the use of hormone therapy does prolong life to a certain degree, it is not nearly as certain as to the difference in anticipated longevity if the hormone treatment is started early in the course of the disease or later in the course of the disease.

Anatomic Location

In Chapter 1, I pointed out that the healthy prostate in the young adult is about the size of a chestnut, and it generally begins to undergo a benign pattern of new growth (BPH) when a man is in his mid-forties. I also likened the prostate to an apple and noted that benign prostatic hyperplasia usually arises in the central part of the prostate gland just under the lining of the prostatic urethra. Carcinoma of the prostate, on the other hand, usually (about 80 percent of the time) arises in the peripheral or outer part of the gland, generally in the true prostate tissue and just under the true capsule of the prostate (the skin of the apple). Since the majority of prostate cancers arrive so near the outside of the gland, it is usually possible to feel them on digital rectal examination of the prostate, as a nodule or a firm, or hard, area (Fig. 5–1). About 20 percent of the time, however, the prostate cancer will arise deep within the gland; in these patients, of course, it is not possible to feel or to diagnose the cancer on digital rectal examination.

In point of fact, the great majority of cancers that are diagnosed in this day and age are diagnosed because an elevated blood PSA level triggers a biopsy of the prostate which then reveals the carcinoma. The great majority of those patients so diagnosed will have a perfectly normal digital rectal examination of the prostate which would trigger no suspicion of prostate cancer. This is because in these patients the PSA blood level becomes elevated long before there are any changes to the prostate gland itself that would suggest cancer.

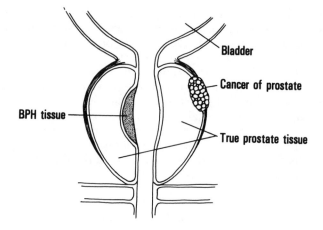

Figure 5–1   *The prostate gland with BPH and cancer. Note that, characteristically, BPH arises in the center of the gland, right around the prostatic urethra, and cancer arises in the periphery of the prostate, where it can often be palpated on digital rectal examination.*

Early and Late Symptoms of Prostatic Cancer

Unfortunately, there are absolutely no symptoms of prostate cancer in its early stages. A possible exception to this statement might be a patient with a very rapidly growing and highly malignant prostate cancer with a rapid spread into the channel of the prostatic urethra so that early in the course of the cancer, symptoms of bladder outlet obstruction would arise. Indeed, whenever an individual who has been voiding with no difficulty has a sudden onset of a weak urinary stream with hesitancy, dribbling, intermittency, and perhaps incomplete bladder emptying, the presence of a rapidly growing carcinoma should at least be suspected. For this reason, I feel that patients who have symptoms of bladder outlet obstruction that have been present only for three months or less should have a prostatic biopsy regardless of how the prostate may feel on digital rectal examination. Not infrequently in these patients, the PSA blood test is elevated thereby confirming the need for a prostate biopsy. However, I believe that patients with a short duration of symptoms of bladder outlet obstruction should be seriously considered for prostate biopsy even in the presence of a normal PSA. The reader should recognize that very malignant prostate cancers do not always make very much PSA, and so the presence of a normal PSA level is by no means an assurance that cancer is not present.

Much more frequently seen are patients with prostate cancer in whom the symptoms of bladder outlet obstruction do not come until relatively late in the course of the disease, after the diagnosis of cancer has been established; the symptoms then result from the very slow growth of the cancer toward and into the prostatic urethra, which causes obstruction to the flow of urine.

A common *late* finding of prostate cancer is the onset of pain in one or more bones that is constant and lasts for two weeks or longer. Such pain is most often in the spine although it might be in the bony pelvis, the low back, the hip, or the bones of the upper legs. When a patient with known prostatic cancer develops these pains, the spread of cancer to the bone must be strongly suspected; when a patient over 50 who is not known to have cancer of the prostate comes to the doctor's office complaining of constant and severe pain in one or more of his bones, prostate cancer that has spread to the bones should be considered in the physician's initial diagnostic approach. A digital rectal examination of the prostate should be carried out promptly to see if any areas suggestive of prostate cancer are noted, and a PSA blood test should of course be done as well. Also, bone x-rays and bone scans (see Chapter 2) should be done. And, of course, prostatic biopsies are necessary before any definitive diagnosis of this disease can be made.

Making the Diagnosis of Prostatic Cancer

At least 80 percent of men in this day and age that are ultimately found to have prostate cancer come to the attention of their doctor because of an elevated PSA blood test. Certainly, an elevated PSA blood test cannot diagnose cancer in and of itself, but it should lead to prostate biopsies in most cases. In the remaining and much smaller group of men in whom prostate cancer is diagnosed, there is usually an abnormal digital rectal examination to suggest the presence of cancer, and this means that palpation of the prostate gland reveals a surface area that is something other than perfectly smooth and of uniform consistency. Areas on the prostate gland that feel irregular or harder than the surrounding areas are not necessarily indicative of cancer, but they very definitely represent an indication for a biopsy of that area with examination of the removed tissue by a competent surgical pathologist whether or not the PSA value is abnormal. The definitive diagnosis of prostate cancer can be made only by the microscopic examination of the removed prostate tissue. If prostatic cancer is to be diagnosed at a time when it is still potentially curable, I believe that a blood PSA test and a digital rectal examination of the prostate should be done annually in all men over the age of 50 and in men over the age of 40 who are African American or who have a first-degree relative (a father or brother) in whom prostate cancer was diagnosed before the age of 60. I feel that all such men who have either an abnormal PSA level or an abnormal digital rectal examination should be referred promptly to a urologist for a consultation and an evaluation.

Obtaining Prostatic Tissue to Confirm the Diagnosis of Prostatic Cancer

Elevations of the blood PSA level to almost any degree can strongly hint that the patient may well have cancer of the prostate. I must emphasize again, however, that prostate specific antigen (PSA) is made by both normal and cancerous prostate cells. Therefore, a large benign prostatic hyperplasia can cause an elevation of up to two or even three times the normal level of PSA. However, when the level of PSA is even higher than this, and particularly when the prostate gland is not particularly enlarged, prostate cancer must be strongly suspected. Thus, a PSA elevation or abnormal areas of the prostate noted on digital rectal exam can lead the clinician to suspect the possibility of prostate cancer. The actual diagnosis, however, cannot be made without obtaining tissue from the prostate, and I believe the most accurate method of doing this is using ultrasound-guided biopsies of the prostate taking as many as ten or twelve biopsies from the various portions of the prostate gland, particularly from the most lateral portions of the gland and from deep within the gland itself.

Certainly, the level of suspicion for prostate cancer can be high when there is a marked elevation of the PSA level (above 10) or when there is a particularly abnormal area of the prostate noticed on digital rectal exam. I should note here that although I feel that prostate biopsies are absolutely essential to confirm the diagnosis of prostate cancer, in fact these biopsies are not always carried out. If a patient is to have an attempt at definitive treatment for the prostate cancer, such as a radical prostatectomy or radiation therapy, then I believe that a prostate biopsy is absolutely mandatory. However, I do not feel it is wrong to place a patient of advancing years (over 75 years of age or thereabouts) in whom the PSA is very elevated and who has a markedly abnormal digital rectal examination on hormonal therapy for the palliation of any symptoms he may have from his prostatic cancer, and I would do this in the absence of a biopsy. These are most unusual situations, but I feel it is worth mentioning them here.

Prostatic Intraepithelial Neoplasia (PIN)

This is a condition that has recently achieved great significance in the management of prostate cancer. Once the prostate gland has been biopsied, obviously the pathologist tells us that the tissue is, hopefully, benign or that there is cancer in the prostate gland. However, there is yet another finding that the pathologist may have to report and that is the presence of Prostatic Intraepithelial Neoplasia (PIN). If this PIN is reported as high-grade, it definitely represents a premalignant lesion, and it may mean that there is already coexisting cancer in the prostate that was not identified at the time of biopsy or that prostate cancer will develop in the future. I would certainly never advocate doing a radical prostatectomy or even radiation therapy on the basis of the finding of this PIN, but when it is reported, I recommend to my patients that they have repeat prostate biopsies within the next couple of months. If these biopsies are negative, I recommend biopsies three or four months after that. In my experience, once a high-grade PIN has been diagnosed, prostatic cancer will inevitably occur at some point. When the PIN diagnosed is reported as low-grade, it is very definitely not a warning of prostatic cancer yet to come, and for patients with low-grade PIN, I recommend following with future prostate biopsies only if they may have a rising PSA level which would dictate such biopsies.

Bone X-rays and Bone Scans

The role of bone x-rays and bone scans in prostatic cancer is simply to determine if the cancer has spread to bone. In other words, bone scans and bone x-rays *only* play a role in the diagnostic study of those patients known to already have cancer of the prostate or those patients with a markedly elevated PSA in whom cancer is strongly suspected or in those patients in whom the prostatic biopsies have been equivocal or perhaps have not been done for some reason.

When cancer of the prostate spreads beyond the confines of the prostate gland the prostate specific antigen blood level is usually markedly elevated (above 20). As already noted, certain very malignant prostatic cancers are so undifferentiated in nature that they are not able to make as much PSA as one would expect from the extent of the cancer, and so this very small group of patients may well have prostate cancer with relatively minimal PSA levels. Whether or not the PSA is markedly elevated, if the patient is thought to be a candidate for curative surgery or radiation therapy, bone scans, and perhaps bone x-rays, may be indicated to be sure that the cancer has not already spread to a bone which would put the patient in a category where definitive treatment such as a radical prostatectomy or radiation therapy would not be indicated because the patient is already beyond the point of cure.

Most of the urologic literature suggests that if the PSA level is under 10, there is virtually no chance that any cancer will have progressed to bone. Some urologists use a PSA of 20 as a cutoff since it is also extremely unlikely that there would be any cancer spread to bone with a PSA of under 20. Both of these numbers may be suspect in the case of high-grade prostate cancers in which the Gleason sum is 8, 9, or 10 (see Chapter 2). In these cases I will still obtain a bone scan regardless of the PSA level before contemplating any potentially curative procedure such as a radical prostatectomy or radiation therapy.

The two principal routes of the spread of prostate cancer are the lymph system to the lymph nodes of the pelvis and the blood stream to various bones of the body, primarily the spine, the pelvis, the hips, and the upper legs. There is no way to tell with certainty if cancer has spread to the lymph nodes except by direct surgical exploration and removal of the nodes with a microscopic examination of these nodes. However, spread to the bones can usually be detected by x-rays or bone scans, and the latter will reveal evidence of the spread to bone several months before the bone x-rays develop the characteristic appearance (see Fig. 2–6). When cancer of the prostate spreads to bone, there is usually an initial partial destruction of that bone followed by the body's normal reparative process which consists of laying down new bone in the area of the destruction. If the bone's destruction is extensive and the reparative process is not, the x-ray appearance of the affected bone will be one of rarefaction or thinning, which may make the bone look like it has punched-out lesions. If the bone destruction is not very extensive, then the reparative process will be the predominant x-ray finding, one of increased bone density. The former lesions are called lytic and the latter are known as blastic, and it should be noted that blastic lesions are far more commonly seen than lytic lesions in patients with prostate cancer that has spread to bone.

Several months before metastatic spread of any kind to bone is detectable by x-ray, bone scans are able to detect the process of regeneration and laying down of new bone in areas that have been the sites of cancer spread. A caveat should be mentioned at this point, and that is that bone scans are not specific to the detection of bone cancer but only reflect the reparative process of bone. This process may also be found in response, for example, to old bone fractures or even to arthritis. Therefore, when bone scans are suggestive of cancer that has spread to bone, correlative plain x-rays of the same bones are taken to see if there is any suggestion that there has been an old fracture or arthritis in those bones. Sometimes a definite determination can still not be made as to whether questionable areas on the bone scan represent cancer spread. In some patients, it is not uncommon to perform hormonal therapy for two or three months, and if the lesions in the bone were indeed caused by the spread of cancer to the bone, a resolution of these areas may be seen as the result of the hormonal therapy. Sometimes, if there is just one bony area involved with the possible spread of cancer and the patient is otherwise considered to be a candidate for definitive treatment (a radical prostatectomy or radiation therapy), a biopsy of the suspicious bone may be done.

Bone scans are done by injecting a radioactive material into an arm vein which then concentrates in bone, and the amount of radioactive material that is taken up by each bone is accurately determined by a counting machine that scans the entire body. Wherever there has been destruction of bone, there will be repair and regeneration, and wherever this occurs, there will be an increased uptake of the radioactive material. The increased uptake of the injected isotope is detected by the counting machine and gives a dense appearance to the scan of those specific bones that are undergoing the reparative process (see Fig. 2–7). Whenever there is an increased radioactivity found over one or more bones in a patient known to have prostate cancer, a strong suggestion of cancer spread to those bones is present.

In the patient known to have cancer of the prostate, then, the role of bone scans and bone x-rays is twofold: first, for the patient thought to have curable prostate cancer, bone scans and bone x-rays are carried out in the expectation that they too will be negative and to make sure that they are, in fact, negative. As already noted, this procedure is usually omitted when the PSA is under 10 (or perhaps under 20) except in the unusual circumstance of a very high-grade and malignant tumor. This use of bone scanning and bone x-rays is one of the steps in the process known as staging a patient to ascertain the presence or absence of cancer spread beyond the confines of the prostate gland.

Second, bone scans and bone x-rays "follow" patients with known prostate cancer to see if and when additional spread of the disease occurs. Such patients may already have had an attempt at curative radical surgery (see Chapter 6), they may be patients who have had radiation therapy in an attempt to cure them, or they may be patients who were seen for the first time when they were already beyond the point of cure. In each of these categories of patients, periodic bone scans and bone x-rays are means of observing and following the progress of these patients, not in the hope of curing them should the cancer appear in one or more bones but to help predict the future course of their illness and to begin additional treatment as promptly as possible once the cancer spread has been determined. In common usage, PSA determinations on a regular basis have replaced the need for these bone scans and bone x-rays in the opinion of many urologists, although a rising PSA level will often result in sending the patient for bone scans or bone x-rays. The higher the PSA level the greater the likelihood of bone cancer from the prostate gland. Generally speaking, the spread of cancer to bone does not usually occur before the PSA level is at least 50.

Abdominal CT scans or an MRI with an endorectal coil may potentially be helpful in determining the presence of enlarged lymph nodes in the patient already diagnosed with prostate cancer. However, these techniques cannot tell the urologist with any degree of certainty whether these enlarged lymph nodes are involved because of cancer or inflammation from some other lesion. In practice, CT scans and MRI scans are not usually done by most urologists when staging a patient to see if the cancer has spread outside of the prostate gland. The use of an MRI with an endorectal coil can be of some help, however, in determining whether the prostate cancer has spread through the capsule of the prostate gland. But this is considered a local extension of the cancer (as opposed to a spread to the lymph nodes) and not a reason why attempted curative therapy with radical surgery or radiation therapy should not be undertaken.

Classification of Prostate Cancer

The statement was made previously that probably as many as 30 percent of men over age 50 have cancer of the prostate, but the vast majority of these men die *with* the disease and not *from* it. Certainly, every urologist can think of many patients alive and well five, ten, even twenty or more years after prostate cancer has been diagnosed. Unhappily, every urologist can also bring to mind a number of patients who lived for only a very few years after the diagnosis of prostate cancer was made. Why the difference? How can one differentiate the "good" cancers from the "bad" cancers?

In an effort to answer these questions, and particularly to plan and implement appropriate therapy for what seems to be almost two different diseases, retrospective studies of large numbers of patients with prostate cancer have been carried out. In these studies, analyses were made of the size of the cancer at the time of diagnosis (one of the criteria used in staging the cancer), and particularly of the microscopic appearance of the cancer as to whether it has the characteristics of low-grade or high-grade malignancy (known as the "grade" of the prostate cancer). This is one of the other criteria used for staging a given cancer.

As noted in Chapter 2, grading prostate cancer is done by most pathologists using the Gleason grading system. Using this system, pathologists assign to prostate cancer (whether obtained by a biopsy or by removal of the entire prostate gland) a number between 1 and 5 on the basis of the microscopic appearance of the architectural pattern of the cancer, with 1 being the least malignant and 5 the most malignant. Most prostate cancers will have more than one pattern of cancer cells, and so pathologists assign a number between 1 and 5 to the predominant cancer pattern in the biopsy (or the surgical specimen) and a second number between 1 and 5 based on the secondary pattern of cancer seen in the specimen. These two numbers (which may be the same) are then added together to provide what is known as the Gleason sum. A Gleason sum of 2, 3, or 4 is considered to be a low-grade cancer; a Gleason sum of 5, 6, or 7 is considered to be an intermediate-grade cancer; and a Gleason sum of 8, 9, or 10 is considered to be a high-grade (highly malignant) cancer.

These two factors, the Gleason sum and the size of the tumor (which can be measured with accuracy at the time the entire prostate gland is removed and can be estimated at the time the biopsies are done on the basis of the number and size of the biopsy specimens having cancer in them), were then studied and compared with the kind of treatment the patient received, whether there were any findings of spread of the cancer, and perhaps most importantly, how long the patient lived after the diagnosis was made. As a result of these studies, cancer of the prostate was classified into stages A, B, C, and D, with subclassifications of each based on the actual size, extent, and location of the cancer as well as the microscopic appearance of the cancer at the time of diagnosis (Fig. 5–2).

More recently, pathologists have revised the staging system to better reflect the clinical situation, and most pathologists (and urologists) now prefer to use the TNM system

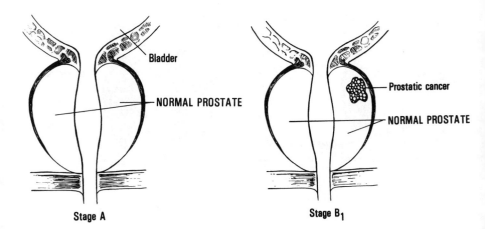

Figure 5–2   THE PROSTATE GLAND SHOWING THE DIFFERENT
STAGES OF CANCER
  Stage A *(T1a, T1b, or T1c). This is the so-called occult stage
of prostate cancer, in which no abnormality of the prostate gland can
be felt or detected on digital rectal examination.*
  Stage B1 *(T2a). This is the stage where cancer is definitely
palpable on digital rectal examination. The cancer is smaller than 1
or 2 centimeters in size and is localized to one side of the prostate
gland.*

instead of the A, B, C, and D system. For purposes of clarity
and for those who may be familiar with one system but not the
other, I will refer to both systems when discussing the staging
and treatment of prostate cancer. In the TNM system, T refers
to the tumor in the prostate gland itself, N refers to nodes of
the lymph system in the pelvis that have cancer in them, and
M refers to metastatic disease presence (the spread of the cancer beyond the pelvic lymph nodes). There are many subdivisions of this TNM system, so it is roughly comparable to the
various subdivisions of the A to D system.
  Stage A cancer (T1) is cancer that cannot be felt by digital
rectal examination in patients, so this examination discloses
an apparently benign prostate gland. It is sometimes diagnosed when a man has surgery for what is thought to be BPH

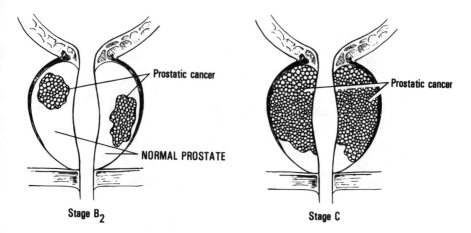

Stage B2 *(T2b)*. *A more extensive form of cancer in which the cancer is larger than 2 centimeters or it is present on both sides of the prostate gland.*

Stages B1 and B2 *(T2a and T2b)*. *Lesions can be detected on digital rectal examination of the prostate gland.*

Stage C *(T3)*. *An extensive prostate cancer where much of both sides of the prostate gland is involved but where it is thought that the cancer has not spread beyond the confines of the prostate gland, although it may have spread through the prostate capsule.*

There is no illustration for a stage D (stage N) cancer because, by definition, a cancer such as this is one in which the prostate cancer has spread beyond the confines of the prostate gland, often to the regional lymph nodes of the pelvis (stage D1 or N) or to more distant sites such as bone (stage D2 or M1).

and the pathologist reports the presence of cancer in the *removed* surgical tissue. Much more commonly, stage A (T1) cancer is diagnosed as a result of an elevated PSA level leading to a positive prostate biopsy.

Stage B cancer (T2) is cancer initially detected as a hard area of the prostate found on digital rectal examination usually as part of a routine physical exam. The digital rectal examination may have been triggered by an elevated PSA blood test but it is considered to be a stage B (T2) on the basis of the physical findings of the digital rectal examination. If the hard or firm area is relatively small (less than 1.5 centimeters) and only in one part of the prostate gland, it is considered to be a stage B1 (T2a) tumor. If the tumor is larger than 1.5 centimeters or is in both lobes of the prostate, it is considered to be a B2 (T2b) tumor.

Stage C (T3) is cancer that on digital rectal examination feels as if it has extended outside the capsule of the prostate.

Stage D1 (N1, N2, or N3) refers to those prostate cancers which have spread to one or more lymph nodes in the pelvis and depends on the volume of cancer in these lymph nodes and the number of lymph notes with cancer in them.

Stage D2 (M1) cancer of the prostate refers to those cancers which have spread to other parts of the body such as the bones or other soft tissues.

Stage A (T1a, T1b, and T1c) Prostatic Cancer

This is a somewhat unusual form of cancer because its diagnosis is sometimes made serendipitously in the absence of any symptoms or physical findings. Its diagnosis can also be suspected by an abnormal elevation of the PSA blood test which triggers a prostatic biopsy. With this stage of cancer, sometimes known as "occult" prostate cancer, the prostate gland feels entirely normal on digital rectal examination. If the patient has an elevated PSA blood test that leads to a prostate biopsy which in turn discloses prostate cancer, then this is known as a stage T1c cancer. Occasionally, these stage A cancers are diagnosed when the patient has a TURP or some other surgical procedure for the relief of bladder outlet obstruction (BPH) and the pathologist then reports that there was cancer found in the removed surgical specimen even though absolutely no cancer was suspected preoperatively on the basis of the digital examination of the prostate. Probably 10 percent of the patients who have prostatic surgery for the relief of the symptoms of bladder outlet obstruction will be found to have this occult prostate cancer. This cancer is divided into A1 (T1a) and A2 (T1b) on the basis of the amount of cancer found in the removed surgical specimen. Pathologists differ on exactly what these amounts are. But, generally speaking, if there are three or fewer microscopic foci of cancer found in the removed surgical specimen, the lesion is considered an A1 (T1a) lesion; if there are more than three microscopic foci of cancer in the removed specimen, the lesion is considered an A2 (T1b) lesion. Also, if the cancer found in the removed surgical specimen is high grade (a Gleason 8, 9, or 10), then the cancer is called an A2 (T1b) lesion even if fewer than three microscopic foci of cancer are found.

These so-called incidental cancers of the prostate that are discovered serendipitously following surgery for the relief of bladder outlet obstruction will vary greatly in their behavior depending on whether the lesions are A1 or A2; the latter kind of cancer is generally more aggressive, suggesting the need for definitive therapy. The A1 (T1a) lesions are often best treated by simply observing the patient and following the patient with PSA blood tests. This is particularly the case for patients who are over the age of 70. Younger patients may be treated with a definitive therapy such as a radical prostatectomy or radiation therapy, or they may simply be followed with sequential PSA blood tests every six to twelve months with any significant rise in the PSA level's suggesting the need for definitive therapy as opposed to observation.

Those patients with stage A (T1) cancers that are detected because of an abnormal PSA elevation with a resulting biopsy of the prostate (stage T1c) are very definitely candidates for definitive treatment since it has pretty well been documented that very, very small amounts of prostatic cancer will not usually bring about enough of a PSA elevation to trigger a biopsy. Reviews of large numbers of patients who have had radical prostatectomies only because of elevated PSA levels, leading to positive biopsies, have confirmed that the overwhelming majority did indeed have significant amounts of cancer in the prostate such that it could be anticipated that the cancers would grow and spread without definitive treatment. Certainly, each patient discovered to have prostate cancer because of an elevated PSA in the presence of a perfectly normal digital rectal examination of the prostate does not necessarily require definitive therapy. The age of the patient is important, and the guide that I always use is the younger the patient, the more the need for definitive therapy because the greater the likelihood that the patient would live long enough for the cancer to spread and kill. As a general rule, I am slow to recommend any definitive therapy for the patient who is over 70 years of age, and I certainly would not recommend any definitive therapy for the patient over 75 years of age. Nevertheless, I am almost always inclined to follow the wishes of my patient about definitive therapy regardless of his age. I can only express my recommendations and my opinions to my patients, but I feel that informed patients are quite capable of deciding what they want to have done to themselves.

For those patients, then, who are stage A (T1a, T1b, or T1c) and who are thought to be candidates for definitive therapy, I believe that the principal options are a radical prostatectomy or radiation therapy. The radiation therapy can take the form of conventional external beam therapy or of brachytherapy in which radioactive seeds are implanted into the prostate gland. This latter procedure is often combined with external beam radiation, and not infrequently, preliminary hormonal therapy is instituted for anywhere from a few weeks to a few months before radiation therapy is done (see Chapter 6). If the patient is to have a radical prostatectomy or either form of radiation therapy and his PSA blood level is over 10, then I generally obtain a bone scan to be sure there is no evidence of any spread of cancer to the bones. If the PSA is less than 10 but the cancer is very high grade (Gleason 8, 9, or 10), I will also get a bone scan. I do not generally see any great merit in obtaining a CT scan or an MRI scan prior to such planned definitive therapy.

In general, I believe that a radical prostatectomy offers a patient the best chance for the most years of life and is clearly superior in the long term to either form of radiation therapy. I recognize that not all physicians will agree with me and certainly there is a definite place for radiation therapy in the treatment of prostate cancer. It is clearly the treatment of choice for those patients who do not wish to have surgery for whatever reason or for those patients who are felt to have other medical conditions that would make such surgery needlessly risky. It is also the treatment of choice for those patients who do not want to run any risk at all of incontinence such as may infrequently occur after radical prostatectomy, and it also is indicated for a patient who wishes to minimize his chances of being impotent as a result of treatment. While radiation therapy does lead to impotence in perhaps half the men receiving such therapy, this is probably somewhat less than the incidence of impotence following radical prostatectomy.

Stage B (T2a and T2b) Prostatic Cancer

Perhaps something under 20 percent of men have this stage of prostatic cancer when it is initially diagnosed. It is to identify and diagnose this stage of cancer that annual digital rectal examinations of the prostate are recommended. These lesions are considered to be curable, and biopsies of the prostate are then carried out following the digital rectal examinations that suggest the likelihood of prostatic cancer. The cure rate of any prostatic cancer will obviously depend on how early in the course of the disease it is diagnosed and treated; this is why I feel so strongly that an annual digital rectal examination of the prostate should be carried out. Relying on the PSA blood test alone is just not satisfactory because, while it certainly will detect many cancers before there are any abnormalities noted on the digital rectal examination, it is also quite true that the PSA blood test can be perfectly normal with prostate cancer, and so that cancer would be undetected in the absence of an abnormal digital rectal exam. Indeed, perhaps as many as 20 percent of prostate cancers that are identified are found in patients with PSAs that are under the often-given upper limit of normal which is about 3.5 (see Chapter 2 for further discussion on PSA values).

Once the palpable lesion in the prostate has been found, a transrectal biopsy should be carried out (see Chapter 2), and the cancer is then staged in much the same manner as was done for the stage A prostate cancers. I believe that treatment options are also very similar to those mentioned for the stage A prostate cancers. The question that regularly comes up concerns the patient with a stage A or stage B (or stage C) cancer of the prostate in whom a radical prostatectomy is planned. Prior to removing the prostate, the pelvic lymph nodes are removed since this is part of the staging procedure to determine how far advanced the cancer is. If removal of these lymph nodes does indeed show the presence of prostate cancer in one or more lymph nodes, this is then known as a stage D1 prostate cancer (a stage N1, N2, or N3 depending on the degree of lymph node involvement). A significant degree of urologic opinion in this country would be that the patient is not curable and the prostate should not be removed. Such patients would then normally be treated with hormone therapy or with observation until there were signs of advancing prostate cancer. However, an almost equal and ever-growing number of urologists in this country feel that patients, even if they have minimal (microscopic) cancer in one or two lymph nodes, may still do quite well by proceeding with the radical prostatectomy and instituting hormonal treatment at or very shortly after surgery. I happen to be a firm believer in this latter school of thought, but I want the reader to recognize that there is no unanimity of opinion among urologists on the subject of what to do when the pelvic lymph nodes show metastatic cancer.

Since radiation therapy is probably not of any curative benefit if any of these pelvic lymph nodes have cancer in them, it is the practice of some urologists to remove these lymph nodes in patients opting for radiation therapy to be sure no cancer is present in them and then to refer the patient for radiation therapy to the prostate gland. It is usually not necessary when the PSA is under 10 or 12 and the cancer is of a low or intermediate grade of malignancy to remove these lymph nodes because in the great majority of patients these lymph nodes will be negative for cancer and the radiation can safely be delivered to the patient even though there is no certainty that the lymph nodes are indeed without cancer.

Stage C (T3 and T4) Prostatic Cancer

A stage C prostatic cancer is more advanced and larger than an A or B stage cancer. On digital rectal examination it is estimated to be a stage C cancer when virtually the entire prostate feels very firm or hard or, alternatively, when the cancer feels as if it has extended behind the base of the prostate up into the seminal vesicles or through the capsule of the prostate gland. At this time a very small percentage of patients are initially seen with a stage C prostate cancer, and indeed, many of the patients thought to have a stage C cancer would be found to have a stage D cancer if surgical exploration of the pelvic lymph nodes were carried out.

Stage C cancer gives no hint of its presence and, by definition, it has not spread outside of the prostate gland (although it may have spread into the tissue immediately surrounding the prostate). Many of the patients who are thought to have a stage C lesion, on the basis of the digital rectal examination, will indeed have significant elevation of their prostate specific antigen levels even though the bone scans and bone x-rays will be negative. In my opinion, a PSA level above 50–100 nanograms per milliliter is pretty strong evidence that a patient in fact has a stage D lesion and not a stage C lesion. Note, however, that lesser PSA values do not preclude the possibility of the cancer's being well outside the prostate gland.

Most urologists feel that stage C cancers are best treated by radiation therapy. My own feeling is that a radical prostatectomy is probably preferable to radiation therapy because I think removing the prostate gland provides better local control of the cancer. By this I mean that it decreases the likelihood of future voiding difficulty and hemorrhage from a large, obstructing, bloody, and malignant prostate gland. If the removed prostate, following a radical prostatectomy, shows extension of the cancer outside of the prostate, there are now very hard and excellent data to show that hormone treatment begun within three months of the radical prostatectomy significantly improves overall survival. Another option when the surgical specimen shows that the cancer extends outside the surgical capsule is postoperative radiation therapy to the site where the prostate used to be.

To sum up, I believe that patients with stages A and B prostate cancers are optimally treated with radical prostatectomy. Stage C prostate cancers may perhaps be preferentially treated with radiation therapy with or without hormone treatment although I still lean toward radial prostatectomy with hormone treatment.

Stage D (N1, N2, N3, and M1) Prostate Cancer

A stage D lesion is one that, by definition, has spread beyond the confines of the prostate gland. If this spread is into the regional lymph nodes, it is considered a D1 (N1, N2, or N3 depending on the number of lymph nodes involved) lesion, and again by definition, one does not speak of curing such patients but rather of giving them the longest possible life taking into account their quality of life and recognizing that this may well be life with coexisting cancer. If the cancer has spread beyond the regional lymph nodes as, for example, to bone, it is considered a D2 (M1) lesion.

Typically, these stage D, or advanced, prostate cancers produce no symptoms at all unless they have already spread to bone in which case they may produce bony pain. Such pain can indeed be quite severe and results from the cancer's invading the bone to a degree sufficient to cause bone destruction. It is a truism among urologists, and should hopefully be so among all physicians, that when a man over the age of 50 comes to a physician with pronounced bony pain in the back, the bony pelvis, the hips, or the long bones of the upper legs, the physician should think very rapidly of the possibility of metastatic carcinoma of the prostate and a digital rectal examination of the prostate should be done as well as obtaining blood PSA levels, bone scans, and bone x-rays if needed. Since the advent of widespread PSA testing, men presenting with stage D cancers are very, very uncommon and probably make up fewer than 5 percent of prostate cancer patients seen by urologists at this point in time. Prior to the advent of widespread PSA testing, as many as 30 to 40 percent of all prostate cancers were initially diagnosed when they were already considered to be stage D.

The role of radiation therapy in stage D1 disease is indeed extremely limited, but there is a definite place for radiation treatment if the pathologist reports that the removed lymph nodes showed no cancer but there was local spread of the prostate cancer through the margins of the surgical specimen following radical prostatectomy. Postoperative radiation therapy may be instituted at that point in time, or it may be delayed until a rising PSA blood level suggests that some cancer remains.

Since all urologists agree that stage D2 lesions are certainly incurable and most urologists feel that D1 lesions may well be incurable, therapies for these advanced forms of prostate cancer are considered to be *palliative* and *not* curative. Certainly, surgery or radiation therapy is probably not going to cure a patient who has *extensive* spread of cancer beyond the confines of the prostate. And, unfortunately, chemotherapy with any of the presently existing anticancer drugs has not been found to be beneficial enough to recommend it as routine treatment. While some specific drugs have achieved temporary relief of symptoms in a small percentage of patients, the use of chemotherapy at this time remains in the experimental or research category. A significant question exists as to the best treatment for a patient who has a markedly elevated prostate specific antigen blood level in the presence of normal bone scans and who has *not* had any surgery to examine and remove the lymph nodes. Should such surgery be done? I feel the prostate specific antigen blood test at this point in time is sufficiently accurate so that its elevation above 100 nanograms per milliliter (and sometimes less) is sufficient proof that the cancer is at least a stage D1. At this point, the philosophy of the urologist regarding the curability of stage D1 lesions will determine whether to recommend simply palliation to the patient or aggressive pursuit of a surgical cure.

If you are wondering about the seeming lack of agreement about the treatment options for the different stages of prostate cancer, remember that the seeming confusion is but a reflection of the fact that there is still much that remains unknown and is yet to be learned about this disease. I personally remain quite convinced that there is definite benefit both in terms of long-term survival (even though often with the presence of existing cancer) and local control by carrying out a radical prostatectomy, with hormonal therapy in certain situations for patients having prostate cancers. Still, this is a quantitative judgment, and the presence of a large amount of cancer outside of the prostate such as might be found with large lymph nodes full of cancer would clearly recommend against proceeding with a radical prostatectomy. In my experience, however, such massive spread of cancer outside of the prostate gland is extremely uncommon.

I think a word about the upper limits of age for patients who are being considered for radical prostate surgery is appropriate. Many urologists feel that a patient over 70 years of age should not have radical prostate surgery because that patient's life expectancy *without* the cancer is not too different from what it might be *with* the cancer. This thinking is based on the fact that the great majority of patients with prostate cancer will live for about ten years in the absence of any attempt to cure the cancer either with radical prostate surgery or with radiation therapy. In general, I tend to agree with this age 70 rule. However, there are many patients who may be over 70 years of age but who are physiologically much younger and in whom a life expectancy of well over ten years may be anticipated. A major consideration in evaluating patients for possible radical prostate surgery is their genetic status; that is, how long did their father, grandfather, or older brothers live? Certainly, those patients who have a genetic predisposition to live to 90 years of age or more would be viable candidates for radical prostate surgery even if over 70 years of age. In short, there is no hard and fast rule on this subject except to say that a patient should have at least ten years of life expectancy absent the prostate cancer in order to be considered for prostate surgery.

A radical prostatectomy is definitely *not* indicated for those patients with stage D2 lesions. This means that there is already evidence of the spread of the cancer beyond the regional pelvic lymph nodes to places such as bone, distant lymph nodes, other organs, or other soft tissue. For these patients hormonal therapy alone is the treatment of choice. For many patients with D1 lesions (where the spread of cancer is noted to be in the pelvic lymph nodes only), in whom aggressive surgical therapy with radical prostatectomy is not felt to be warranted, either because of the patient's wishes, the urologist's philosophy, or the patient's general state of health, hormonal therapy is also the treatment of choice. However, the best time to begin this hormonal therapy is unclear and there is a considerable difference of opinion among urologists on this point.

PSA Following Radical Prostatectomy

Once a radical prostatectomy has been done for stage A, B, or C (T1, T2, T3, or T4) lesions, the PSA should drop to undetectable or virtually undetectable levels. If it does not do so within a month or so after surgery, the presumption is that there is still residual cancer in the patient. Usually, this cancer is within the area where the prostate gland used to be, and radiation therapy to that area is often recommended. This will often bring the PSA down to undetectable levels. About 25 to 30 percent of patients in whom the PSA went to undetectable levels following the radical prostatectomy will have a gradual rise in PSA within four or five years after the time surgery was performed. This usually means that there is now some prostate cancer that has recurred. There is no test that will tell with certainty exactly where this cancer recurrence is, so the recommended treatment may be radiation therapy to the area where the prostate used to be (sometimes an ultrasound-guided transrectal biopsy of the area will be done) or hormonal therapy if it is felt that the recurrent cancer is elsewhere in the body. Sometimes the recommended treatment may be both radiation and hormonal therapy. The goal with any therapy is to get the PSA level as close to undetectable as possible and to keep it at that level as long as possible.

Hormonal Therapy and Other Medical Therapy for Stage D Prostate Cancer

About 90 percent of prostate cancers are androgen dependent; this means that the growth of these cancers is enhanced by the influence of male hormones (androgens). The presence of these androgens (predominantly testosterone), which circulate normally in the male, actually aids and abets the growth and spread of the prostate cancer. The other 10 percent of prostate cancers are nonandrogen dependent; this means that the growth and rate of spread of these prostate cancers bears no particular relationship to the presence or absence or quantity of male hormones circulating in the body.

Since the vast majority (90 percent) of patients with stage D prostate cancer have cancers that are androgen dependent, it is a fact that reduction of the circulating androgen (testosterone) levels to near zero has been proven to slow down the rate of growth of cancer and to make the patient feel better. It must be reiterated, however, that this form of treatment is purely palliative and is definitely not curative. In other words, it tends to slow down the progression of the prostate cancer and it probably prolongs life to a degree, but it very definitely must not be considered as a potentially curative treatment.

There are several ways of markedly reducing the level of male hormones (testosterone) in the body to therapeutic levels. The most obvious is the removal of both testes, called bilateral orchiectomy. This is clearly the most cost-efficient manner and it is, obviously, not reversible.

The other principal method of lowering circulating testosterone levels has become extremely popular in the last several years because it avoids the mental trauma to a man of having his testes removed. It is not cost effective, however, since the administration of these injectable medications can run to $6,000 or $8,000 per year, a cost that is presently covered by most insurance policies but in an era of cost containment it is questionable as to whether these injectable medications will be reimbursable in the future. It has been found that certain hormones act on the male pituitary to initially cause an outpouring of additional testosterone. This might seem paradoxical, but after about a week of this action on the pituitary, these injected hormones cause the testosterone level to drop to zero, which is about the level achieved when both testes are removed. The reason for this effect is somewhat difficult to comprehend, but the action itself is highly reproducible and valid.

These injectable hormones that act on the pituitary gland are known as luteinizing hormone-releasing hormones (LH-RH), and they are given in the form of injections that are administered by a doctor or a nurse. These injections can be given monthly, or they can be given at intervals of three or even four months because the LH-RH medications are available in long-term dosage formats. The cost, as noted, is quite prohibitive in whatever form the medication is given, and the medication must be given indefinitely because if it is stopped, the serum testosterone level will again rise. Recently, it has been shown that in some patients the intermittent use of these LH-RH injectable hormones can achieve results that are just as good as the regular administration of these injections, but this will vary from patient to patient. Because of the very high cost of these injections and of the inconvenience of requiring injections at regular intervals, a bilateral orchiectomy is without any doubt considered to be the "gold standard" for palliation of prostate cancer, although the injections of these LH-RH hormones are certainly an acceptable alternative for those patients who refuse bilateral orchiectomy.

Since the goal of hormonal therapy in the treatment of advanced prostate cancer (stage D) is to decrease the circulating level of male hormones to zero or as close to zero as possible, it should be noted that the adrenal glands do in fact produce some very small amounts of male hormone and there is some evidence to suggest that suppression of the adrenal androgens with direct antiandrogen therapy achieves a better overall result for these patients than can be achieved simply by suppressing the testicular androgens which is done either by bilateral orchiectomy or the use of LH-RH hormones. Suppressing the adrenal androgens along with the suppression of testicular androgens is referred to as "combined androgen blockade." The use of this combined androgen blockade is by no means universal or even widespread because the evidence that it significantly prolongs life as compared with the suppression of testicular androgens only is somewhat spotty, and it appears that at best it might prolong life for only a few months beyond that which is achieved by suppressing testicular androgens alone.

In any case, the use of combined androgen blockade is certainly a well-recognized treatment for prostate cancer and the adrenal androgens can be suppressed with any of three antiandrogens available in this country. These are flutamide (Eulexin), bicalutamide (Casodex), and nilutamide (Nilandron). Of these three medications, the bicalutamide (Casodex) would appear to be the preferred form of therapy because it can be given in a one-tablet once-a-day dosing regimen and it has fewer side effects than the other forms of therapy. Ketaconazole should probably also be mentioned as another of the antiandrogen drugs, but for various reasons, it has not been used nearly as widely as the drugs just mentioned. Finally, it should be noted that estrogen therapy has been used for many, many years to suppress circulating androgens and it will indeed do this to a very satisfactory level. However, the estrogen levels needed to achieve this androgen suppression to a therapeutic level have been found to cause very deleterious effects on the cardiovascular system and so this use of estrogen therapy in the treatment of advanced prostate cancer has been abandoned for the most part.

A major question does frequently come up regarding the palliative treatment of advanced (stage D) prostate cancer with hormonal therapy, whether the hormonal therapy consists of testicular androgen suppression or combined androgen blockage. This is a question of the optimum time to begin such therapy. The early landmark studies of the late 1930s and 1940s did conclusively demonstrate that androgen deprivation (at that time it was done with orchiectomy alone) prolonged the life of patients with stage D prostate cancer and also improved the quality of life remaining to the patient.

Various studies since then have attempted to determine whether these salutary effects from the hormonal therapy are optimized by starting it at the time that the cancer has been determined to have spread (and thus become stage D) or after

the patient has definite symptoms from the spread of the cancer such as bone pain. The answer now appears to be pretty
clear, at least in those patients who have had a radical prostatectomy and in whom minimal involvement of the regional
lymph nodes with prostate cancer was noted to be present.
Clearly, these patients have had the longest survival when for-
mal treatment has been started early either by bilateral
orchiectomy at the time of the radical prostatectomy or by the
prompt postoperative commencement of LH-RH hormonal
therapy by injection. The optimum timing of hormonal therapy for patients who have *not* had surgery but in whom
advanced prostate cancer is very likely on the basis of a significantly rising and high PSA level is still open to question. However, it would appear that early hormonal therapy is better
than delayed hormonal therapy on the basis of experience
with patients who have had radical prostatectomy and early
hormonal therapy.

There is no argument about the prompt starting of hormonal therapy when a patient has definite evidence of the
spread of the prostate cancer to bone. The question really
comes up when a patient with diagnosed prostate cancer has
a PSA that has risen to 40–50 or more which would suggest
that the cancer may well have spread outside of the prostate
gland and for whatever reason the decision had already been
made that the patient is not to be a candidate for either radical prostatectomy or radiation therapy. There are really no
hard data to indicate when hormonal therapy should be started in such cases. However, starting the hormonal therapy earlier rather than later appears to make the most sense although
the side effects of such therapy (hot flashes and fatigue) are of
sufficient concern to many patients that they choose to delay
hormonal therapy until their cancer has begun to cause symptoms such as bone pain. I certainly lean toward starting hormonal therapy earlier rather than later because it does appear
to make more sense, but the timing of this therapy is dependent in large measure on a patient's wishes and his PSA level
since there are very few hard data to support the benefit of
early hormonal treatment.

There are some problems with hormonal treatment. The
long-term use of hormonal deprivation as a therapy, whether
by surgical removal of the testes or by LH-RH injections, leads
to gradual loss of bone that can ultimately result in osteo-

porosis. This is not to make the point that hormone deprivation therapy should not be carried out, but it must be realized
that at some point in time, if a patient has been hormonally
deprived for many years or even several years, osteoporosis
may well occur leading to bone fragility and potential bone
fractures.

Unfortunately, sooner or later, hormonal therapy usually
fails and the patient is then in a condition known as "hormone
resistant." This condition is determined by a continuing rise in
the PSA level even in the presence of the hormonal therapy or
by the obvious progression of metastases to structures such as
bone. At this point in time, there is no further therapy that has
been proven to extend a patient's life beyond the year or two
that might remain once a patient becomes hormone resistant.
However, a potentially very exciting new treatment may significantly increase a patient's survival and that is a combination of estramustine, which is given orally, with Taxotere,
which is given intravenously. Early clinical trials show that this
may indeed significantly increase survival but it is as yet in the
category of "very promising agents under study." In other
words, the final word is not yet in, but doctors working with
this combination of drugs are very hopeful that it will at last
represent a significant breakthrough as regards an increase in
survival time in patients who have become hormone resistant.
There are many agents under investigation and in common
use. Estramustine alone has not been very beneficial but in
combination with various agents (such as Taxotere) it has
shown to be of some benefit. When a patient does become hormone resistant, I believe that referral to an oncologist for one
of the many clinical trials now under study may well prolong
a patient's life and certainly can make whatever time remains
more comfortable. The efficacy of any drugs used once a
patient has become hormone resistant can be monitored and
measured by the PSA level. A decline in the PSA level by 50
percent is associated with an increased life expectancy
although the ideal result of treatment would be a normaliza-
tion of the PSA level or at least a decline of 75 percent.

Survival Statistics

As we have seen, cancer of the prostate can almost be considered to be many different diseases because the activity of

the cancer varies enormously from patient to patient. However, it does appear quite clear that the larger the size of the cancer and the higher its microscopic grade (Gleason sum) at the time of diagnosis, the poorer is the outlook for a cure or a long-term survival. For those cancers that are extremely small and of very low microscopic grade (stage A1 or T1a), the survival will be about the same as it would be for an individual without prostate cancer. These very small, often microscopic, foci of prostate cancer represent the kind of cancer that patients die *with* and not *from*, and it is this specific kind of cancer (A1 or T1a) that I am referring to when I say that up to 30 percent of men over age 50 have prostate cancer.

Probably the most important single parameter in determining cure or long-term cause-specific survival is the Gleason sum. The reader should understand that cause-specific survival may be quite different from survival because the former implies that the death is caused by the prostate cancer whereas simple survival (without the specific cause mentioned) refers to death from any cause. Obviously, in the age group under discussion many people may die of heart disease or some cancer other than prostate cancer before they may die from prostate cancer. In the very best of institutions following radical prostatectomy a patient with a low Gleason sum (2 to 4) can anticipate a 95 percent ten-year cause-specific survival. This figure drops to 88 percent when the Gleason sum is 5 to 7, and it drops further to 64 percent when the Gleason sum is 8 to 10. Remember that all of the cause-specific survival data is just that and does not address posttreatment PSA levels. All patients who have prostate cancer are followed—at least once a year and often more frequently—with PSA blood tests whether they have been treated with radical prostatectomy or radiation or watchful waiting. While the majority of patients who have had a radical prostatectomy have PSA levels that remain undetectable indefinitely, this is not the case with all patients. So, when cause-specific survival data are presented, it does not necessarily mean the patient is totally free of cancer. Rather, it means that these patients are clinically well although they may not have undetectable PSA levels.

The PSA number is also an independent variable that is helpful in predicting cause-specific survival. The outcomes following radical prostatectomy for patients with PSAs that are 10 or less are far superior to those for patients with PSAs greater than 20 at the time of radical prostatectomy. The PSA may be considered an indirect measurement of tumor volume, and the higher the PSA, the greater the volume of cancer that is present.

Another important variable in trying to predict long-term cause-specific survival or cure in prostate cancer patients is the ploidy of the cancer itself. "Ploidy" is the abbreviation for "nuclear DNA ploidy pattern"; this is the pattern of the total DNA content of the nuclei of a given sample of tissue as plotted on a graph that is known as a histogram. The acronym DNA stands for deoxyribonucleic acid, which is a complex protein found in all cells. The process by which these graphs or histograms are plotted on the basis of the DNA content in the nuclei of the cancerous tissue cells is called "flow cytometry," a highly sophisticated and technically complex procedure that is based on the fact that most tumor cells have abnormal amounts of DNA. The diploid pattern of DNA is clearly the most common that is found in patients with prostate cancer, and this type of ploidy pattern produces the best results in terms of cure or long-term cause-specific survival.

For patients with a diploid tumor pattern and a stage D1 cancer (with spread to the pelvic lymph nodes), the ten- to fifteen-year cancer-specific survival is 90 percent or greater when they are treated with radical prostatectomy and hormonal therapy (either removal of the testes or injections of an LH-RH agonist). Few patients with diploid cancers treated in this way die of their disease. For patients with T2 and T3 disease (stage B and stage C), the survival outcome for those with diploid tumors is much better than for those with nondiploid tumors. In fact, very few of those diploid patients who undergo radical prostatectomy will be dead from prostate cancer in a ten-year follow-up. While it is true that the majority of patients who have prostate cancer confined within the prostate gland will have a diploid type of tumor, it is also true that those cancers which spread to the regional lymph nodes often have a nondiploid pattern (tetraploid or aneuploid), and those patients having nondiploid tumors do not do quite as well as those patients having diploid tumors.

Patients with A2 (T1b) lesions are usually diagnosed by a prostate biopsy which is triggered by an elevated PSA blood level. Some few such patients with A2 (T1b) lesions are diagnosed following a TURP with examination of the removed tissue. Regardless of how diagnosed, these tumors (A2, or T1b) are certainly significant cancers, and when treated with radical prostatectomy, the ten-year cause-specific survival is about 95 percent and the 15-year cause-specific survival is about 92 percent.

In treating patients with a stage D1 prostate cancer (with spread to the pelvic lymph nodes), the prevailing thought until recently has been that these patients are incurable and any contemplated radical prostatectomy should be aborted. Because of compelling data that have been accumulated for the last ten or more years from several leading institutions in this country, the pendulum has swung back to the point where patients with stage D1 disease (cancer that has spread to the pelvic lymph nodes) may still be curable or at least have a long-term cause-specific survival if a radical prostatectomy is carried out and accompanied by hormone deprivation, either by removal of the testes or with LH-RH agonist injections. The cause-specific survival of patients who had cancer that had spread to the pelvic lymph nodes and who were treated with radical prostatectomy and hormone ablation was 91 percent at five years, 79 percent at ten years, and 60 percent at fifteen years. These figures include patients with diploid and nondiploid tumors. As noted, patients with diploid tumors clearly did better than patients with nondiploid tumors, and it is interesting to note that the increased cause-specific survival (for both diploid and nondiploid tumors) when the hormone ablation was added to the radical prostatectomy was most noted beyond ten years after radical prostatectomy.

In fact, cause-specific survival up to ten years is the same whether the radical prostatectomy is combined with hormone ablation or not; but cause-specific survival increases significantly from ten years on and extends toward fifteen years if hormone ablation is combined with the radical prostatectomy. The reader should note that in discussing these D1 cancers (where the spread of cancer has gone to the pelvic lymph nodes), the reference is to minimal cancer in the regional lymph nodes that is detected by microscopic examination of the lymph nodes. Where there is massive spread of cancer to the regional lymph nodes such that the lymph nodes are enlarged to many times their normal size, a radical prostatectomy is not generally carried out. It should be noted, however, that it is extremely rare to find such massive involvement of the pelvic lymph nodes with prostate cancer.

Finally, there are interesting data that are available at this point in time suggesting a difference in cause-specific survival between palpable cancer and nonpalpable cancer, that is, prostate cancer that is discovered on digital rectal examination of the prostate and prostate cancer that is discovered because of an elevated PSA blood level. Both of these will trigger a prostate biopsy that is positive for cancer. In other words, we are discussing PSA-detected versus digital rectal examination–detected prostate cancer. If a patient has a PSA-detected cancer (stage T1c), cause-specific survival at ten years after radical prostatectomy is about 99 percent. Fifteen-year follow-ups are not yet available because the PSA has not been in common usage for that long. For those patients undergoing radical prostatectomy because of a palpable lesion in the prostate gland (stage B1, or T2a), there is a ten-year cancer-specific survival rate of 95 percent, and for patients with even more extensive palpable cancer in the prostate (stage B2, or T2b), the ten-year cause-specific survival is 93 percent. So there does appear to be a definite survival advantage to patients who have their prostate cancers detected by PSA as opposed to digital palpation of the prostate gland. It is generally felt that the detection of prostate cancer by PSA levels alone provides at least a five-year clinical lead time in the detection of clinically significant disease as compared with the detection of prostate cancer by digital rectal palpation of the prostate gland.

I must hasten to point out to the reader at this point that the cause-specific survival data provided throughout this section represent the very best such data from our best institutions. The number of patients who have had radical prostatectomy and on whom the foregoing data are based is an extremely large number, and therefore the results are statistically valid and very accurate. Excellent results such as noted above may be found in many of our leading institutions in this country although results such as these may not necessarily be found universally.

The survival data just presented, although excellent, will undoubtedly lead many readers to the obvious question: Why shouldn't the cause-specific survival rate be 100 percent when the lymph nodes show *no* evidence of cancer involvement and all other tests are similarly negative for the presence of prostate cancer? This is, of course, a central question to survival data for any cancer, but the less than 100 percent survival is because of the unfortunate fact that there may indeed have been a spread of cancer outside the confines of the prostate gland (but not to the lymph nodes) and this spread has been a microscopic one that is not detectable. However, when the pelvic lymph nodes have no evidence of any cancer in them, the ten-year and beyond survival data indeed approach 100 percent (for diploid tumors), and this does indeed illustrate the excellent results that can be obtained in the treatment of low and intermediate Gleason sum prostate cancer by a radical prostatectomy.

Alternative Therapies

It constantly amazes me how very intelligent patients, told that they have prostate cancer, seek alternative remedies that could best be described as "fringe" treatments. While it is certainly true that some prostate cancers will grow so slowly that it would appear that a patient may be cured, the fact remains that for patients with a life expectancy that is much more than ten years, no forms of therapy other than radical prostatectomy, external beam radiation therapy, implantation of radioactive seeds into the prostate, or a combination of these modalities has ever been proven to cure people or to prolong survival with a good quality of life. I can readily understand the reluctance of a patient, particularly a young man, to undergo surgery or even radiation therapy because of the potential complications of either and his desire therefore to seek other treatments that are totally unproven and totally unscientific. And I fully recognize that we physicians by no means have all of the answers, and there may well be certain very helpful treatments that many physicians tend to disregard. Certainly, it is very possible that there may well be various herbal treatments that can palliate, if not cure, prostate cancer.

One such herbal remedy that has had some success in bona fide clinical trials is known as PC-SPES, and it is used in patients who have become hormone resistant, a phase that usually heralds the end of life. The PC stands for prostate cancer and SPES is Latin for "hope." The PC-SPES is a group of eight herbs that have been used with resulting decreases in PSA levels although without any definite objective signs of clinical improvement. There are risks from toxicity when using this PC-SPES, and the cost can run as high as $500 per month. I do not believe that this PC-SPES is going to provide the magic bullet for the cure of advanced prostate cancer, but the results of some of its trials would indeed suggest that alternative (and complementary) forms of therapy should not be dismissed lightly.

Prevention of Prostate Cancer

Although all proven treatments for prostate cancer have already been mentioned in this chapter, it is certainly possible that there may also be ways to prevent or delay the onset of prostate cancer. There are numerous ongoing studies in this country and abroad using various chemopreventive agents, and there are certainly many ongoing studies in molecular and cellular biology, genetics, and experimental carcinogenesis that may help with such chemoprevention of prostate cancer. Four of the stated goals of such chemoprevention are inhibition of carcinogens (agents that might precipitate prostate cancer), intervention for persons at genetic risk of prostate cancer (those patients who have a father or brother who developed prostate cancer prior to age 60), treatment of precancerous lesions (such as prostatic interepithelial neoplasia, a precancerous condition that is found on prostate biopsies), and evaluation and interpretation of various leads from dietary epidemiology. Experimental studies in animal tumor models, for example, have identified several nutrients that have potential as chemopreventive agents.

The use of such cancer prevention requires chemopreventive agents with virtually no toxicity. Vitamins D and E have periodically been thought to have cancer inhibition properties. Vitamins A and C have similarly been thought at various times to have properties that enable them to inhibit carcinogenesis. A diet that is low in fat has very definitely been shown to prevent prostate cancer in rats; whether this is translatable to humans remains to be seen. Many long-term trials will be required before any definite statements can be made regarding bona fide methods for preventing prostate cancer or delaying the onset of such cancer in men. Chemoprevention trials with finasteride (Proscar), isoflavonoids, retinoids, and selenium are underway. Certain chemicals from soy products have been thought to decrease the risk of prostate cancer. The list goes on and on, and hopefully the day will come when prostate cancer will be preventable. As of now, however, there is no proven or documented way to prevent prostate cancer and certainly there is no sort of diet change or dietary addition known to cure prostate cancer.

Vaccines

Ultimately, it is hoped that a vaccine may be developed that will prevent prostate cancer. At present, no such vaccine exists. However, there are at least two companies presently manufacturing vaccines that one day might be utilitized to treat patients who already have prostate cancer. In theory, these vaccines could be used for any patient with prostate cancer, but at this time they are being employed only to treat patients who have failed either radical prostatectomy or radiation therapy and who have a rising PSA level. These vaccines, it must be emphasized, are highly experimental and are by no means in regular clinical use except as part of research protocols. The principle of these vaccines is based on trying to stimulate a patient's own immune system in the hope that this will intensify that patient's resistance to the cancer and enable that patient to conquer his cancer. Blood is drawn from such patients, and a specific type of white cell is removed from this blood and then treated in such a way that when it is injected back into the patient it might serve to stimulate the immune system. I must emphasize that this is still very, very experimental and not in any way to be considered as an existing form of treatment for cancer of the prostate.

6

Minimally Invasive Techniques, True Surgical Procedures, and Radiation Therapy

Question: What did the fortieth president of the United States have in common with almost 400,000 other U.S. men?

Answer: In 1987, all of these individuals had surgery to relieve the symptoms of benign prostatic hyperplasia (BPH); the vast majority of these operations (including that of the president) were done using the transurethral approach by an operation known as TransUrethral Resection of the Prostate (TURP).

In very recent years the treatment of benign prostatic hyperplasia has undergone very significant changes, and these changes have come about because of the medical (pharmacologic) treatment for BPH (see Chapter 4) as well as numerous other innovative approaches to the surgical treatment of this condition. A major driving force pushing these newer surgical procedures has been the massive effort at cost containment, and many of these newer procedures have enabled the patient to spend less time in the hospital thereby saving considerable amounts of money. Some of these procedures even allow for the treatment of BPH in an office setting (outpatient). Obviously, all methods of treatment of BPH are not equally efficacious, and most of the newer ones just have not been around long enough to have established any sort of track record for durability beyond just a few years. This means that although these newer methods may achieve satisfactory results in the short term, there is just not enough known about the long-term results and possible complications to be able to say unequivocally that these newer procedures are as good as the "gold standard" which is the TURP.

It is my intent to discuss in this chapter these various procedures in some degree of detail so the reader may better understand them. I recognize that not all readers may want to read this chapter since it may be more technical than some of you may like and because it isn't always pleasant to read about surgical procedures that may be carried out on oneself. Nevertheless, for those interested in knowing precisely what will be done to them when they have prostate surgery, I hope that this chapter will provide the answers. I also feel it is appropriate in this chapter to make some general statements about radiation therapy procedures for cancer of the prostate, including the implanting of radioactive seeds into the prostate; how these procedures are done; and their short-term and long-term side effects. Finally, I think it appropriate to go into some detail about the surgery done for removal of the testes (bilateral orchiectomy) since this procedure is done, or at least recommended, for the treatment of prostate cancer that has already spread outside the limits of the prostate gland.

Minimally Invasive Techniques for the Treatment of Benign Prostatic Hyperplasia

Minimally invasive techniques generally refers to procedures that can be done in an office setting with minimal discomfort to the patient and usually without the need of any spinal or general anesthesia. There are really only two such techniques in common usage that come under this category, and these are the use of heat (microwave thermotherapy) and the TransUrethral Needle Ablation (TUNA) technique. The first of these procedures, also known as heat therapy, is done in an office setting, usually with only a local anesthetic jelly placed into the urethra, and it involves the placing of a catheter into the urethra such that the heating element of the catheter is positioned within the prostatic urethra. There is also a cooling element within this catheter so that even though the prostate gland itself is heated to 60 to 65 degrees Celsius, the urethra is kept cool and protected from any damage. The resulting coagulation effect on the prostate gland results in a retraction of the prostate gland away from the urethra and, therefore, a widening of the urethral channel through which the urine flows. There are several systems on the market using this form of microwave thermotherapy and the equipment that has probably received the best reception from many urologists is the Targis System (Fig. 6–1).

With this form of treatment for BPH a patient is usually treated in an office setting for a period of an hour or two under a local anesthetic that is squirted into the urethra; the patient is then able to leave and return to his home. There is usually enough swelling within the prostatic urethra immediately following the procedure that voiding can become difficult, and so an indwelling catheter is necessary for a few days. However, the patient is able to go home with this catheter in place. Bleeding is usually relatively minimal. Most patients are able to return to their normal activities within a few days. The principal advantage of this form of treatment for benign prostatic hyperplasia is that it can be performed in an office setting thereby resulting in very significant cost savings because it does not require an operating room, the presence of anesthesia personnel, intravenous sedation, or general or spinal anesthesia. It comes under the heading of "minimally invasive treatment" of the BPH because it can be done in an office setting.

The other minimally invasive treatment is the Trans-Urethral Needle Ablation (TUNA) of the prostate, and this is done by introducing radio frequency energy into the prostate gland through needles that are placed transurethrally into the gland. A cystoscope-like instrument is introduced into the urethra, and from the end of this instrument two needles are advanced into the substance of the prostate gland which is then treated by this radio frequency energy. This results also in a type of coagulation necrosis of the prostate gland thereby enlarging the channel through which the urine flows and alleviating some of the symptoms of benign prostatic hyperplasia. Although TUNA has been promoted as an office procedure, in the hands of many urologists it does require anesthesia standby for intravenous sedation or a prostatic nerve block which is not always easy to perform. For these reasons the

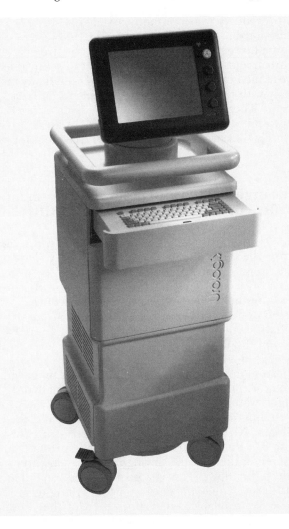

Figure 6–1 *The Targis System for microwave thermotherapy. Pictured here is the delivery apparatus; not pictured is the catheter that is attached to this apparatus and which is then inserted into the patient's urethra. Also not pictured here is a suitable table on which the patient would be lying. (Photograph courtesy of Urologix, Minneapolis, Minnesota.)*

TUNA procedure, while certainly a viable means of treating BPH, has not achieved very widespread usage.

To sum up regarding these minimally invasive procedures for the treatment of BPH, I would say that they are at least as effective as medical therapy (see Chapter 4) and many patients are happy with the results of these treatments, at least in the short run. These treatments have not been around long enough to say whether the long-term results are satisfactory, but certainly they are very good forms of treatment for selected patients.

True Surgical Procedures for the Treatment of Benign Prostatic Hyperplasia (BPH)

These procedures are considered to be "true" surgical procedures because they are almost uniformly done in an operating room setting under either a spinal or a general anesthesia or at least with intravenous sedation that usually requires anesthesia personnel. These procedures include vaporization of the prostate, laser treatment of the prostate, TransUrethral Incision of the Prostate (TUIP), TransUrethral Resection of the Prostate (TURP), and "open" surgery of the prostate (Fig. 6–2).

Vaporization of the prostate is carried out by means of a transurethral approach using a type of roller ball that delivers a very high wattage to the prostatic urethra and the prostate gland resulting in vaporization of the prostate and the prostatic urethra. No tissue is removed with this procedure, but the result is a diminution in the size of the prostate and an enlargement of the channel through the prostatic urethra via which the urine flows. This is a good procedure and at least the short-term results are satisfactory. The long-term results are not as yet available, but vaporization of the prostate is widely done at this point in time and certainly must be considered to be a satisfactory procedure.

The use of lasers in the prostate gland has had mixed reports depending on the type of lasers used. Most of the earlier types of laser treatments have now been abandoned because patients had pretty severe voiding discomfort for a good three months following surgery. However, the use of the interstitial laser appears to be very promising and patients are

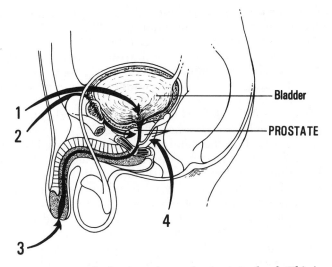

Figure 6–2   *Surgical approaches to the prostate gland. This is a lateral view of a man, through the midportion of his body, and shows the four procedures that truly can be called surgical procedures on the prostate gland: (1) the suprapubic approach; (2) the retropubic approach; (3) the transurethral approach; (4) the perineal approach.*
     Note that of these approaches only the TURP is used frequently. The other open surgical approaches are very, very infrequently used.

quite happy with this. With the interstitial laser, fibers are advanced through the urethra directly into the prostate gland thereby avoiding any damage to the urethra itself. The interior of the prostate gland is coagulated by means of the interstitial laser fibers while the urethra is preserved. It is the destruction of the urethra itself that is responsible for most of the discomfort postoperatively when other types of laser procedures are used. This interstitial laser procedure is probably the most widely used laser procedure at this time.

Another type of laser procedure in use is the Holmium laser procedure. This produces very salutary results except for the fact that it removes chunks of prostate tissue (unlike other laser procedures where the tissue is congealed) and then sometimes it can be very difficult to remove those chunks of prostate tissue from the bladder. Efforts are being made to develop a procedure for the morcellation of these chunks of prostate tissue, and when this is done, the Holmium laser may become the standard means of laser treatment.

Finally, a new and as yet experimental form of laser treatment uses a KTP laser with an extraordinarily high wattage; it is this high wattage that is not yet commercially available. With this procedure the tissue is vaporized and the patients have very few complaints following surgery. Ultimately, this may prove to be the laser procedure of choice.

As regards all of the different laser procedures, it can be said that they do indeed increase the flow rate and decrease the symptom score, but many of them have their own complications and their long-term efficacy is still somewhat questionable because they have not been used for that many years. Certainly, laser treatment of the prostate is a valid form of therapy that is here to stay and will probably produce better and better results as better equipment becomes available.

The transurethral incision of the prostate is an old procedure and a resectoscope is used for it. The urologist makes deep incisions into the prostate in the five and seven o'clock positions from just inside the bladder neck all the way out to a point just before the external urethral sphincter (Fig. 6–3). That is all—two simple incisions with no attempt to remove any of the obstructing prostate tissue. Most urologists who are enthusiastic about this operative procedure feel that it produces results comparable to those offered by the TURP and that it also has a comparable length of hospital stay and comparable postoperative bleeding. All agree that it is primarily suitable for small prostate glands and undoubtedly its biggest, and perhaps its only, advantage is that it leads to retrograde ejaculation (see Chapter 8) much less frequently than the TURP. Absent or reduced ejaculation occurs in about 10 to 25 percent of patients who have this operation; this compares favorably with the 50 to 70 percent retrograde ejaculation occurrence after the TURP, a problem of real concern to some patients.

TransUrethral Resection of the Prostate (TURP)

In talking about surgical procedures for the relief of benign prostatic hyperplasia, the procedure that immediately

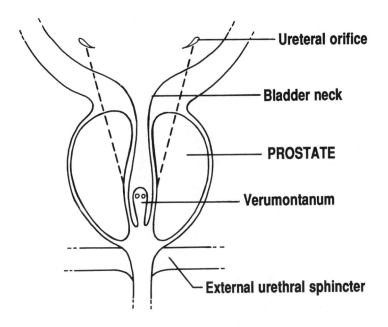

Figure 6–3   *TransUrethral Incision of the Prostate (TUIP). The dotted lines indicate the two positions (five and seven o'clock) in which deep cuts are made beginning just below the ureteral orifices in the bladder and extending outward to a point just inside the verumontanum. These incisions go all the way through the prostate adenoma as far as the surgical capsule of the prostate.*

comes to mind is the TURP. This procedure has been in widespread usage since before World War II although it has continuously been improved and refined. There is no question that it must be considered the gold standard for the treatment of BPH, and it is the procedure against which all of the other procedures mentioned in this chapter must be measured. Its efficacy and its long-term results are well known, and it is in comparison with these excellent long-term results that one is forced to say regarding all of the other procedures for the treatment of BPH that their long-term results are not yet well known.

    To understand in some detail exactly what is done during a TURP (and in the open operative procedures yet to be described), a few of the anatomic facts that were pointed out in Chapter 1 need to be recalled. Each of the surgical approaches to BPH (the TURP and all of the open approaches) is based on the same principle: all of the tissue that is *within* the surgical capsule must be removed and the true prostate tissue and the true capsule of the prostate are left. Please note that for the minimally invasive procedures as well as for the vaporization and the laser procedures, no attempt is made to remove all the tissue that is within the surgical capsule. With these procedures the tissue is vaporized, coagulated, congealed, or whatever thereby enlarging the channel through which the urine flows. These procedures are obviously, therefore, different from the TURP or any of the open procedures yet to be described.

In removing all of the tissue that is *within* the surgical capsule, it should be understood that the prostatic urethra itself will be removed and will be replaced naturally by a new lining that will grow down from the bladder. Remembering the analogy of the apple with the core removed in which the hole through the apple represents the prostatic urethra, you will recall that it is just under the lining of the prostatic urethra that the BPH begins to grow. If it grows in an inward direction, it will obstruct the channel of the prostatic urethra. It may, and usually does, also grow in an outward direction, giving an enlarged feel to the prostate on digital rectal examination. As the BPH grows in an outward direction, it compresses the true prostate tissue between itself and the true capsule of the prostate.

Between the expanding growth of the BPH and the true prostate tissue, there is a plane which is called the surgical capsule. As used here, *plane* refers merely to the point at which two separate tissues (the BPH and the true prostate tissues) touch one another. The surgical "capsule" is not a capsule at all but simply the name given to the interface between the BPH tissue and the true prostate tissue. It may be visualized as the relationship between a piece of Scotch tape and a piece of cloth on which the tape is resting. The surgical capsule would be the interface of the sticky side of the tape and the cloth. The surgical treatment of BPH involves removing all of the tissue that is inside of the surgical capsule, leaving behind the true prostate tissue and the true capsule. The tissue that is being removed is only the BPH itself and it includes the lining of the prostatic urethra (Fig. 6–4). The only difference between the TURP and the open procedures for BPH is the approach to the BPH tissue itself, but all of the procedures effectively do the same thing.

Anesthesia in Prostate Surgery

Spinal anesthesia, an injection into the spine that blocks pain but leaves the patient awake is the preferred anesthesia since it ideally combines total absence of pain and complete relaxation of the patient with virtually no postoperative lung problems. It is often difficult to achieve all of these benefits with a general anesthesia, but for the patient who has abnormally low blood pressure or certain types of heart problems, general anesthesia may be best since spinal anesthesia may cause acute and sudden lowering of the blood pressure which could present a problem. Spinal anesthesia is also often avoided in patients who have had back surgery or spinal cord injuries.

Transurethral Prostate Surgery

The modern era of transurethral prostate surgery (also known as transurethral resection of the prostate or TURP) goes back to the 1950s. In the intervening years the technique and the instrumentation has been polished and refined so that the operation today is as successful and as excellent as any major surgical procedure in terms of low death rate, few complications, and excellent surgical results. The operation is done through the urethra with an instrument that is similar to the cystoscope and is called a resectoscope (Fig. 6–5). When the instrument is positioned within the prostatic urethra, obstructing BPH tissue is cut away, beginning in the center of the prostatic urethra and working toward the periphery of the prostate gland until the surgical capsule is reached. At this point all of the BPH tissue has been removed and only the true prostate tissue is left.

When the resectoscope has been introduced through the urethra and into the bladder, it is possible to note the type and extent of prostatic enlargement that is present. This enlargement will consist of enlargement of the middle lobe, enlargement of the two lateral lobes, or enlargement of all three lobes. The principle of the transurethral approach to prostatic surgery is to trim away the obstructing prostatic tissue starting from the inside of the prostatic urethra and working toward the outside of the prostate gland. Imagine putting an instrument inside a very narrow and obstructed core of an apple and then, working from the inside of the core in an outward direction toward the skin of the apple, trimming away the pulp of the apple until the core is enlarged to the point that there is no pulp obstructing the channel.

Sometimes, this may involve trimming away the obstructing BPH growth until just a very thin rim of tissue remains just under the true capsule of the prostate. At other times, trimming away the obstructing new growth of prostate (the BPH) may only require the removal of a few pieces of BPH tissue. Although enlargements of the middle lobe are probably the most common cause of prostatic obstruction and can cause the most severe symptoms of obstruction, it is interesting that in terms of actual size or amount of obstructing tissue, the middle lobe is usually quite small and often less than 20 grams in weight. Middle lobe enlargement cannot be detected on digital rectal examination of the prostate gland. Lateral lobe prostatic enlargement, on the other hand, can be very great

Figure 6–4   THE PROSTATE GLAND BEFORE AND AFTER SURGERY TO RELIEVE BENIGN PROSTATIC HYPERPLASIA

A. An extensive growth of benign prostatic hyperplasia tissue stretching the true prostate out toward the periphery of the prostate gland and severely encroaching on the prostatic urethra.

B. The prostate gland following surgery. Note that all of the benign prostatic hyperplasia tissue has been removed, leaving a large prostatic urethra through which urine flows.

C. Within several weeks following surgery, the true prostate gland contracts so that the prostatic urethra once again has a configuration such as it did before the BPH started to grow. The compressed true prostate tissue was able to resume its normal configuration, filling the vacancy left by the removal of the BPH tissue. Note that although this figure most closely illustrates what happens after a transurethral resection of the prostate gland, the principle and the end result are not too dissimilar to the principle and the end result of any of the open operations for BPH.

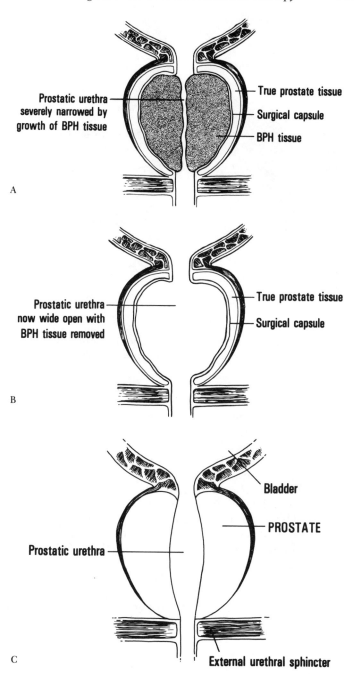

Prostatic urethra severely narrowed by growth of BPH tissue

True prostate tissue

Surgical capsule

BPH tissue

A

Prostatic urethra now wide open with BPH tissue removed

True prostate tissue

Surgical capsule

B

Bladder

PROSTATE

Prostatic urethra

External urethral sphincter

C

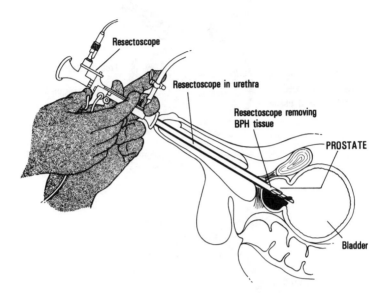

Figure 6–5   *TransUrethral Resection of the Prostate (TURP),
showing the surgical instrument (the resectoscope) in the urethra
and in the bladder as the surgeon removes pieces of tissue from the
prostate gland.*

and extensive in terms of the amount and weight of tissue that
needs to be removed in order to relieve the obstruction. It is
these massive lateral lobe enlargements that can yield 50 to
100 grams or more of BPH tissue that must be removed.

During the course of the surgical procedure, which takes
perhaps an hour or an hour and a half, many blood vessels,
both arteries and veins, are cut across; so, bleeding can be considerable. This is the reason it is necessary to have an irrigation system that ensures the continuous supply of fluid
flowing through the resectoscope and into the bladder, keeping the surgical field clear of blood while the urologist is trimming away the obstructing BPH tissue. During this
continuous irrigation the bladder fills every twenty to thirty
seconds so it becomes necessary to periodically stop the continuous flow, empty the irrigating fluid from the bladder

through the resectoscope, and start again. Some urologists prefer to use a type of resectoscope that permits continuous drainage of the irrigating fluid, thereby obviating the need to periodically stop in order to empty the bladder. The pieces of prostate tissue (BPH) that have been removed up to that point leave the bladder through the resectoscope along with the irrigating fluid. Since it is not possible to clamp and tie off the blood vessels that are cut during the course of surgery, as is done with open operative procedures, these blood vessels must be fulgurated, or "cooked," with a coagulating electrical current that the urologist is able to apply directly to the bleeding blood vessels. The skill of the urologist is of the utmost importance in the outcome of a transurethral prostatic resection in terms of removing all of the obstructing BPH tissue without injuring or destroying normal prostate tissue, being able to control by fulguration the many blood vessels that invariably bleed during surgery, not injuring any of the anatomic areas that control urinary continence, and not damaging the normal bladder neck which could lead to a bladder neck contracture (see Chapter 8).

Following removal of all of the obstructing prostate tissue, a Foley catheter is placed into the patient's bladder and the balloon is inflated to keep the catheter in place for one or more days while the very small blood vessels within the prostatic urethra that cannot be coagulated seal themselves off and stop bleeding (Fig. 6-6). The catheter also allows continuous irrigation of the bladder for a day or so after surgery in order to minimize clot formation as a clot would act as a foreign body within the bladder and cause painful bladder spasms. Clots would also act to impede the drainage of urine to the outside. The drainage from the catheter is usually clear enough by the day following surgery (and sometimes even the day of surgery) so that the catheter can be removed. Microscopic blood, and perhaps even visible blood, will normally persist in the urine for a number of weeks following surgery until the prostatic urethra is entirely healed.

Although the results of this type of surgery are usually excellent, you must remember that when surgery by any approach for the relief of BPH is done, the true prostate tissue is left behind and so also is the cause (which is not totally understood) of the original growth of BPH tissue. Therefore, it must be anticipated that a certain number of individuals will

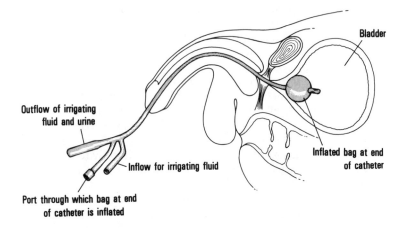

Bladder

Outflow of irrigating
fluid and urine

Inflow for irrigating fluid

Inflated bag at end
of catheter

Port through which bag at end
of catheter is inflated

Figure 6–6   *Immediately after a TURP, a Foley catheter is placed
through the urethra and into the bladder. This figure shows the
catheter in place following the TURP. Note that a similar catheter
would be placed, at least briefly, following just about any of the procedures described in this chapter for the treatment of BPH (other
than pharmacologic treatments).*

have a regrowth of BPH tissue, necessitating another operation. Obviously, the younger a man is when he has prostate
surgery, the greater the likelihood of a regrowth because he
will presumably live for many years after the initial operation.
But it must be remembered that this is an age-related phenomenon. An 80-year-old man having his first TURP is highly unlikely to ever need another one whereas a 45-year-old
man will very likely need another such operation if he lives
long enough.

It should be noted that a TURP is a very difficult operation to perform and one that requires considerable skill on the
part of the urologist. Certainly, it is far more difficult to perform than any of the minimally invasive procedures or any of
the laser or vaporization procedures. It also, generally speaking, produces superior results to those of any of the other procedures in terms of relief of symptoms and increase in voiding
flow rate. The trade-off, however, is that a hospitalization is
required with its necessary disadvantages which particularly
include significantly greater costs.

Open Surgical Approaches for the Treatment of Benign Prostatic Hyperplasia

These open operations for BPH are rarely done nowadays, but they are included in this chapter in the interest of completeness and because there are some few situations in which they are still performed.

The Suprapubic Approach

The suprapubic approach (the word *pubic* refers to the pubic bone) to the prostate (suprapubic prostatectomy) is through the lower abdomen, making an opening into the bladder. The prostate is reached with a hand inside the bladder, with the index finger's advancing through the bladder neck and down into the prostatic urethra. There are two very similar operations: the "blind" suprapubic approach and the visual, or open, one.

The blind approach, so-called because the entire operation is done by feel alone and not under direct vision, was developed in 1896 by Peter Freyer. In 1909 Thompson Walker originated the visual, or open, suprapubic prostatectomy which allowed the operating surgeon to see the surgical field directly and to control bleeding by placing stitches into the bladder neck. The two procedures, however, are really very similar.

Blind Suprapubic Prostatectomy The principal advantage of this type of operation is that it requires only a minimum of surgical expertise and a minimum of special equipment. It can also be done with something less than excellent abdominal relaxation and exposure of the surgical field; therefore minimal anesthesia expertise is required. The primary disadvantage of this technique is the difficulty in controlling bleeding since the bleeding vessels are never visualized. In this day and age of surgical excellence, however, there really are no specific indications for this type of operation except perhaps if the patient is being cared for in an area where there is an absence of surgical assistance and a paucity of specialized urologic instruments. This procedure must not—repeat not—be done when the patient is known to have cancer of the prostate since it is frequently not possible to separate and remove the BPH

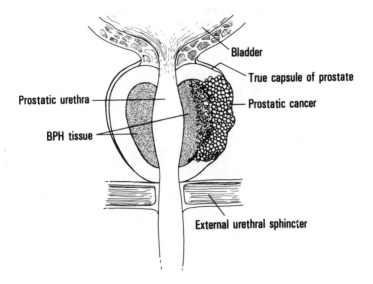

Figure 6–7   *A prostate gland with both benign prostatic hyperplasia and cancer. Note that the cancer tends to grow in an inward direction from the periphery where it arose. In growing in this inward manner, it grows right through the plane of the surgical capsule, thereby making it extremely difficult or even impossible to enucleate, or "shell out," the BPH tissue via any of the open surgical approaches. For this reason, a patient who is known to have prostate cancer, and in whom the only indication for surgery is relief of voiding difficulties (with no attempt at a cure of the cancer), should only have the transurethral approach to the prostate gland.*

tissue from the underlying true prostate because of the strong possibility that the cancer has spread from the true prostate (where it arose) directly into the BPH tissue (Fig. 6–7). Attempts to remove the obstructing BPH tissue may well result in tearing and ripping the prostate gland right through its true capsule since the usual cleavage plane of the surgical capsule is no longer present because of the cancer. For this same reason, *none* of the open surgical procedures should be used for the treatment of BPH if cancer is known to be present.

With the patient lying flat on his back on the operating table, an incision from the navel to the pubic bone is made and

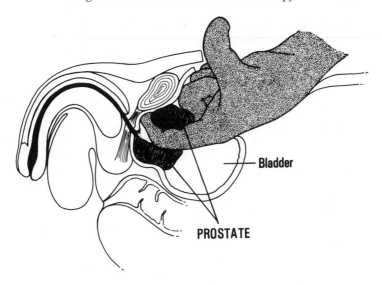

Figure 6–8   *The blind suprapubic surgical approach to the prostate gland, in which the surgeon's finger is inserted into the bladder and then into the prostatic urethra before starting to remove the BPH tissue.*

extended down through the layers of the abdominal wall until the bladder, which has been distended with water put in through a Foley catheter, is exposed. The bladder is opened and the index finger is placed through the bladder neck and down into the prostate urethra. Then that index finger breaks through the urethra in an upward direction at the level of the far end of the prostate, and the removal of the BPH begins (Fig. 6–8). Recall that in this blind suprapubic approach, as in all of the surgical approaches to BPH, the principle of the surgery is to remove *all* of the tissue that is within the surgical capsule. When the index finger has broken through the prostatic urethral lining as well as the BPH, it will stop at the plane between the BPH and the true prostate tissue (the surgical capsule) because the BPH splits easily before the upward pushing motion of the index finger while the true prostate is more resistant and does not easily yield. Once the index finger has found the plane between the BPH and the true prostate tissue, the surgeon slips the finger around in that plane, embracing an arc of 180 degrees first on one side and then on the other until all of the BPH tissue is separated from the underlying true prostate.

With this operative approach it is not possible for the surgeon to visualize the bladder neck very well; and it is certainly not possible to visualize any part of the interior of the true prostate once the obstructing tissue has been removed. It is therefore not possible to identify any bleeding vessels. Control of bleeding, which can be profuse, is usually done by placing a large gauze pack into the inside of the true prostate gland where it is left for several minutes. This will usually stop the bleeding or reduce it to a minimum. The bladder is then closed with stitches and a large catheter-like tube is brought out of the bladder directly through the lower part of the abdomen while a smaller Foley catheter is placed into the bladder through the urethra. With two catheters to drain the blood and the urine, the likelihood of blood clots' plugging both catheters is minimized.

I generally prefer to remove the bladder tube that is coming through the abdominal wall once the drainage from both catheters is relatively free of blood. With the urethral catheter still in place, the opening into the bladder where the removed catheter had been closes spontaneously in a day or two after which the urethral catheter is removed. It is generally several days before the urine is quite clear of blood, both catheters are removed, and the patient is able to go home.

Visual, or Open, Suprapubic Prostatectomy The same reasons for doing a blind suprapubic operation apply to the visual procedures; and the reasons for *not* doing the blind operation apply as well. When the visual operation is done, the incision into the bladder is made much closer to the bladder neck so that it is possible for the surgeon to see the bladder neck and to control bleeding after the obstructing prostate tissue has been removed. Further, with the visual operation, it is also possible to do a neater and cleaner repair of the denuded bladder neck in the area from which the obstructing prostate tissue was removed. In all other ways, however, the operation is similar to the blind operation. In practice, the vast majority of all operations that are now done using the suprapubic approach are done in a manner that permits the surgeon to see the bladder neck and to accomplish reasonably good control of bleeding. The postoperative course is the same for the open as for the blind approach. It should also be noted that a more recent variation of the open approach allows for the placing of sutures at the five and seven o'clock positions at the bladder neck which helps to control bleeding.

The reader may fairly wonder why a suprapubic prostatectomy is done at all in view of the obviously increased morbidity involved with this procedure and in view of the excellence of both the TURP and the very definite acceptability of the other methods for treating BPH. The answer is really quite simple. Suprapubic prostatectomy is indeed very, very rarely done. It is mainly done when it is felt that the prostate gland is just too large to manage transurethrally and this means something over 75 grams. Very few patients will have prostates of this size, but prostates of this size certainly do occur at times. The other possible reason for doing a suprapubic prostatectomy is if there are large stones in the bladder and it is felt that the best way to remove these is by opening the bladder. Once the bladder is open, it is tempting to go ahead and do a suprapubic prostatectomy although it is perhaps equally good logic to close the bladder and do a transurethral resection of the prostate. Finally, when patients have bladder diverticulae that need to be surgically removed, it is necessary to open the bladder and so a suprapubic prostatectomy can be considered at this time as well.

The Retropubic Approach The retropubic approach (retropubic prostatectomy) was first utilized in 1909, but it was not established on a sound and firm basis until 1945 when an English surgeon, Terrence Millen, popularized the procedure. This approach, as with the suprapubic approach, is primarily indicated when a massive amount of obstructing prostate tissue is present, an amount that is felt to be too large for the transurethral operation. Note that this operation does not give the same excellent access to the bladder as the suprapubic approach does. The retropubic approach, as well as the suprapubic approach, is also indicated for those patients whose inability to flex their hips precludes the lithotomy position that is necessary for the transurethral approach.

The advantages of the retropubic approach are that it permits very excellent exposure of the prostate gland and of the bladder neck and thereby facilitates accurate control of bleeding after the obstructing tissue has been removed. The bladder itself is not opened with this approach, and there is no need for a catheter coming through the bladder wall following surgery as is necessary with the suprapubic approach. The disadvantages of the retropubic approach are primarily that very specialized surgical instruments are needed and the exposure of the prostate gland can be extremely difficult in obese men or in those with a particularly narrow or deep bony pelvis.

The operation is usually performed with the patient flat on his back. The same up and down incision is made in the lower abdomen as is made when using the suprapubic approach. The incision is carried through the layers of muscle in the abdomen; then the area *under* the pubic bone is cleaned so that the entire surface of the prostate gland is exposed. Because the surgical exposure is primarily behind and under the pubic bone, the operation is known as a *retropubic* prosta-tectomy. Once the area under the pubic bone and directly over the prostate itself has been visualized, an incision is made in the true capsule of the prostate just below the bladder neck. The incision is deepened through the true prostate tissue to the plane marking the junction of the true prostate tissue from the growth of BPH tissue (Fig. 6–9). This plane is known as the surgical capsule which was described before, and when it is reached, it is readily recognized. The enucleation, or "shelling out," of the BPH tissue is then done all the way around the circumference of the prostate gland; the tissue inside this plane is removed with the surgeon's finger and a long, curved scissors.

The reader should note that this is very similar to the suprapubic operation except that with the latter the enucle-ation, or shelling out, of the BPH tissue begins in the channel of the prostatic urethra and moves in an outward direction, whereas with the retropubic operation it begins at the outside of the prostate gland and moves in an inward direction. With both operations the end result is the same. In both operations all of the BPH growth is removed along with the lining of the prostatic urethra, since it is the inner lining of the BPH growth. Bleeding in the retropubic operation is controlled by placing stitches in the bleeding areas which are easy to visual-ize; therefore the postoperative complication of bleeding is less common than with the suprapubic approach. The bladder neck is trimmed and "neatened," the catheter is advanced

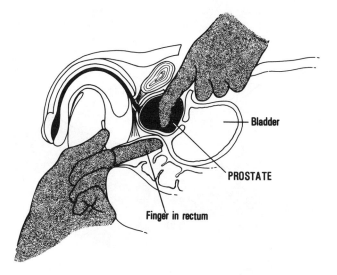

Figure 6–9 *The retropubic approach to the removal of BPH tissue, in which the surgeon's finger does not enter the bladder but goes directly through the true capsule of the prostate in order to remove the BPH tissue. This finger in the rectum elevates the prostate and facilitates the surgery.*

through the urethra and into the bladder and left there for a few days, and the incisions in the prostatic capsule and in the abdominal wall are closed.

Retropubic prostatectomies are very uncommonly done in this day and age although it certainly is an excellent operation and can logically be the procedure of choice for urologists who have developed great expertise with this operation when it is used for patients with very large prostate glands.

Perineal Prostatectomy

This operation is done through the perineum which is the area between the scrotum and the anus. In 1903 the present operation using this perineal approach for relief of BPH was devised by Dr. Hugh Young (Fig. 6–10). This surgical

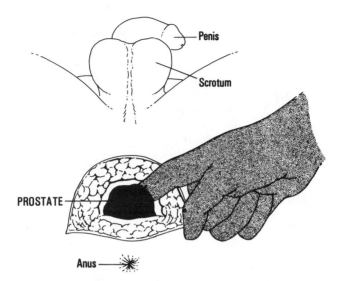

Figure 6–10 *The perineal approach to the removal of BPH tissue, in which the incision is made in the area between the patient's anus and scrotum and the prostate gland is approached from below.*

approach has very few advantages over the other approaches and in fact it is almost never used for the treatment of BPH.

Rarely Used and Investigative Methods for Treating Benign Prostatic Hyperplasia

Stents

In very infrequent situations such as when a patient has a very short life expectancy but the use of a catheter is not acceptable for one reason or another, metal stents made of a nickel-titanium alloy can be placed transurethrally into the prostatic urethra. These stents expand after they are placed to increase the size of the prostatic urethra and permit voiding. It is not good to use them when the patient's problem is a large middle lobe, and in general, they are considered only in very specific and selected patients because they are intended to be temporary and they are not infrequently the cause of considerable patient discomfort.

High-Frequency Focused Ultrasound (HIFU)

This is an experimental procedure in which ultrasound waves are used to destroy prostate tissue. It is as yet an investigational treatment and is not available commercially; whether it ever achieves widespread usage remains to be seen.

Alcohol Injections

Quite recently some urologists have been experimenting with the injection of pure alcohol into the prostate gland transurethrally via needles that go directly into the prostate gland. This has been found in animal studies and in some very few human studies to cause a shrinkage of the prostate gland. Whether this procedure becomes commercially feasible and available remains to be seen, but it is something that seems to have real potential and should be followed up.

Psychological Considerations

There is undoubtedly a great deal of anxiety, and at times even fear, connected with almost any kind of physical disease even if it does not require surgery. When the required form of treatment *does* involve a surgical procedure, the anxiety and particularly the fear increase dramatically. Diseases of the prostate gland are of especially great concern to most men, and if the disease requires a surgical treatment, it can inspire fearful thoughts of a most unhappy nature. As with many things that promote fear, it is the unknown and the out-and-out myths and old wives' tales that are most to blame for such concerns and anxieties. I cannot stress strongly enough how very important it is for a thoughtful and caring physician to explain to his patient exactly what is involved in the contemplated surgical procedure to treat BPH, what the complications of the surgery may be, what the convalescence period is like, and of the utmost importance, what does *not* happen to the patient and to his sex life.

A very common and extraordinarily widespread myth about prostate surgery (for benign disease) is that once a man has had it, his sex life is finished. This absolute falsehood is undoubtedly passed along in locker rooms, bars, and late-night poker games wherever men congregate. There is no question about the fact that a patient undergoing surgery will do better and have a smoother convalescence if he is relatively free of anxieties or fears of any kind, but particularly of those related to the surgery. When the surgery is for BPH, the common and often expressed fears about the "end of my sex life" can be very effectively countered by the physician who will take the time and the interest to do so. Since much of erectile dysfunction (impotence) is psychic in origin, it is probably accurate to say that the patient who goes into surgery feeling quite certain he will be impotent as a result of the surgery will often be exactly that. The fact of the matter is that a patient's sexual abilities following BPH surgery will usually be precisely the same as they were before surgery, with the caveat that most patients having surgery for BPH are in their sixties, seventies, or even older and some will already have a greater or lesser degree of erectile dysfunction *prior* to the surgery.

It is a very convenient and easy thing for a patient, following surgery, to blame his sexual problems on the operation itself rather than to admit to himself that the problem is "his own fault." It is also not unlikely that an elderly male who has lost interest in having a sexual relationship with his wife will see fit to attribute this loss of interest to the surgery. In point of fact, the overall statistics show that about 10 to 20 percent of men who claim they were perfectly potent prior to surgery say that they are unable to achieve erections following surgery for benign prostatic hyperplasia. The reasons for this are varied, and whether the reason is a functional or an organic one is a moot point. The point is, however, that the great majority of men who are potent preoperatively will remain so postoperatively regardless of the specific technique used to treat the benign prostatic hyperplasia.

Positive reinforcement of these facts prior to surgery truly works wonders in alleviating patient concerns about their ability to continue with a sex life after surgery. The urologic surgeon usually understands, perhaps far more than other surgeons, that patients who are having surgery on the prostate gland need to be given an opportunity to ventilate their fears and concerns. For those patients who are uncomfortable about initiating these discussions, the urologist will often bring up the subject and speak to the patient's concerns. There are many excellent urologists practicing in this country, and most of them are as caring and thoughtful about their patient's needs and anxieties as they are excellent in the performance of the surgical procedures. I believe that if you, as a patient, find yourself in the care of a urologist, however technically excellent he may be, who is less thoughtful and less caring about your worries and your anxieties than you would like him to be, it is only logical for you to ask your primary care physician to refer you to another urologist.

Watchful Waiting

As I have indicated more than once in the foregoing pages, I do believe that if a patient's only problems are those of symptoms related to bladder outlet obstruction, the patient should be allowed to determine if and when he wants treatment for these symptoms. I have followed patients for months and years with such symptoms waiting for them to determine if and when they wanted surgery; this procedure is known as watchful waiting. Many patients will have a slight amelioration of their symptoms over a period of time, some will remain unchanged, and probably most will have a gradual worsening of their symptoms. When I speak of watchful waiting, I do not mean benign neglect; rather, I like to follow these patients on at least an annual basis, and sometimes more often, and at such visits I will ask them about their symptoms, check their urine for signs of infection, get an ultrasound of the bladder to make sure they are emptying their bladder reasonably well, and if there is a question of incomplete bladder emptying, I will get an ultrasound of the kidneys to make sure there is no evidence of any back pressure on the kidneys. Finally, I will get a blood creatinine level to make sure there has been no decrease in kidney function. I will usually do these various studies at approximately yearly intervals, but I will encourage my patient to come in any time if he notices a worsening of his symptoms.

Some Final Thoughts about Different Approaches in Treating the Symptoms of Benign Prostatic Hyperplasia

As I noted in Chapter 4, if a patient's *only* problem is the symptoms of voiding difficulty such as getting up frequently during the night, having a weak urinary stream, voiding frequently, and so on, I am almost always inclined to let a patient decide if and when he wants to have treatment for this condition. When a patient does choose to have treatment, I like to start on one of the alpha blockers such as doxazocin or terazocin (Cardura or Hytrin) or I may put the patient on finasteride (Proscar) if he has a very large prostate gland. If the patient is symptomatically improved with medical treatment, I believe he should be allowed to stay on it for as long as the treatment works and as long as the patient is willing to continue taking daily medication. If the medication does not work to the satisfaction of the patient or if it worked initially and no longer seems to help *or* if the patient has *objective* findings of bladder outlet obstruction (a large amount of postvoid residual urine, recurrent bladder infections, decreasing kidney function, blockage of one or both kidneys, and so on), then clearly some form of surgical treatment is necessary whether of the minimally invasive type or not.

At this point I will almost always perform a pressure/flow study (see Chapter 2) so as to be quite certain that the problem is a bladder outlet obstruction and not a primary bladder problem that would not be helped at all by any procedure on the prostate gland. Assuming that the diagnosis of bladder outlet obstruction is confirmed by the pressure/flow study, the question then is whether one of the minimally invasive treatments is preferable or one of the procedures requiring the use of an operating room such as the laser procedure, the vaporization, the TUIP, or the TURP. It is generally my practice to discuss the various options with a patient and sometimes patients have very definite opinions about what they want.

All other things being equal, I believe that the TURP remains at this point in time the gold standard both in terms of short-term and long-term salutary effects, and I tell this to the patient. Not infrequently a patient will have read about a procedure such as the vaporization or the use of a laser and will request this procedure, and that is perfectly reasonable. A lot will also depend on which types of procedures the patient's insurance covers and whether the patient wants to be treated as an outpatient or an inpatient. Finally, if the patient is a poor health risk, one of the minimally invasive procedures would certainly be preferable. There are many factors to consider, and I think it is perfectly reasonable to discuss these with a patient and equally reasonable for the urologist to steer the patient to the type of therapy that the urologist has found to be preferable through experience. However, it is perfectly proper and reasonable for you, the patient, to ask your urologist why he prefers the particular approach that he has recommended, and it is also proper to ask him as many other questions as you may have so you are completely satisfied with your urologic surgeon and with the planned procedure.

Assuming that you have confidence in your primary care physician who has referred you to this urologist and assuming that your urologist is either board certified (by the American Board of Urology) or board eligible (he or she has taken the requisite training to be certified but has perhaps not been in practice quite long enough to have taken the oral part of the certification examination), I think you should feel comfortable with your urologist. However, you should always realize that there are many excellent urologists in this country, and if you are not happy, for whatever reason, with the individual to whom you have been referred, you should certainly feel free to ask your primary care physician to refer you to someone else. You should also never hesitate to ask your urologist if he or she is board certified or board eligible. Alternatively, you can look the urologist up in the *Marquis' Directory of Medical Specialists* which is updated frequently.

Surgery for Cancer of the Prostate

The preferred treatment, in my opinion, for cancer of the prostate is the radical or total removal of the prostate gland when the patient's disease is at a stage where a long-term survival or cure can be anticipated and there are no contraindications to such surgery. This means that the patient has at least ten years of life expectancy absent the prostate cancer and no severe medical problems that would significantly increase the risk of the surgery.

The operation for cancer of the prostate is fundamentally and completely different from any and all of those operations already described for the treatment of BPH because the *entire* prostate gland is removed (Fig. 6–11). When the entire prostate is removed in an attempt to cure prostate cancer, the bladder is brought down into the pelvis and the bladder neck is stitched to the stump of the urethra at the point where the prostate gland was detached from it. In this manner, the gap where the removed prostate had been and the continuity of the lower urinary tract is reestablished. Obviously, a radical, or total, prostatectomy (these terms are synonymous) is completely unrelated to the several operative procedures for the relief of BPH that we have just discussed. In these other operations, the term *prostatectomy* is often used, but it is a misnomer since the procedure that is done for BPH is a removal (or a vaporization or a desiccation) of *only* that portion of the prostate gland that is obstructing the flow of urine (the BPH) leaving behind the true prostate tissue and the true capsule of the prostate.

There are two distinct and different surgical procedures that are used when a radical or total prostatectomy is done. The first, and the one which I much prefer, is the retropubic approach. This operation is known as a radical, or total, retropubic prostatectomy, and it is very different from the operation that is done for BPH that is known as a conservative, or simple, retropubic prostatectomy. However, it does use the same surgical approach to the prostate, and that is from behind and under the pubic bone. The second surgical procedure for prostate cancer is known as a radical perineal prostatectomy. It uses the same approach (through the perineum) as the conservative, or simple, perineal prostatectomy that is very, very rarely used in the treatment of BPH.

The primary advantage of a retropubic approach to a radical prostatectomy is that it permits the removal and examination of the lymph nodes of the pelvis, and these are the lymph nodes to which prostate cancer tends to spread sooner or later depending on how long the cancer has been present. These lymph nodes are known as the obturator and the iliac lymph nodes, and it is these nodes that are removed and examined microscopically as part of the staging procedure to see if a prostate cancer has already spread to them. The lymph nodes can be examined and the results reported within about twen-

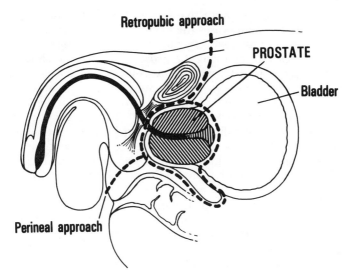

Retropubic approach

PROSTATE

Bladder

Perineal approach

Figure 6–11   *The principle of radical or total prostatectomy (removal of the prostate) for the treatment of prostate cancer. The dotted lines indicate that the approach can be retropubic or perineal. The dotted lines also indicate that the entire prostate gland and the seminal vesicles (included within the dotted lines) are removed in this type of operation.*

ty minutes, using an examining technique known as a frozen section. As we have seen, there is no consensus among urologists about whether to proceed with a radical prostatectomy if there is evidence of cancer spread to any of the lymph nodes. My point is simply that unless the lymph nodes are examined prior to removing the prostate gland, the presence or absence of tumor in these lymph nodes cannot be known, and these lymph nodes are most readily examined when the retropubic surgical approach is used. I should add at this point that a considerable body of knowledge has arisen by now concerning the likelihood of any cancer's having spread to lymph nodes, and this is based on the microscopic grade of the prostate as seen on biopsy (the Gleason sum), the preoperative PSA blood level, and the stage of the cancer as determined by the preoperative digital rectal examination.

Taking all these predictive factors together, some urologists feel that in many cases the likelihood of any lymph node spread is so minimal that removal of these lymph nodes is not necessary prior to removing the prostate gland. In such cases, the principle reason for doing a retropubic prostatectomy as opposed to a perineal prostatectomy is no longer apparent and either route would be satisfactory. In practice in the United States, between 80 and 90 percent of the radical prostatectomies done annually are in fact done via the retropubic approach. I should also mention that the recent popularization of laparoscopic techniques in urology has made it possible to remove the lymph nodes in the pelvis through four very small incisions in the abdomen (Fig. 6–12). On the basis of the frozen section reports, the urologist may proceed with the radical prostatectomy, but the point is that those surgeons preferring to do a radical prostatectomy through the perineal route can remove the lymph nodes laparoscopically.

The retropubic approach to the prostate for a radical prostatectomy is precisely the same as for the retropubic approach for BPH. A long up-and-down incision is made in the midline of the abdomen from the navel to the pubic bone. After the lymph nodes have been removed for study by the pathologist and a determination has been made to proceed with the removal of the prostate gland, the space underneath the pubic bone is cleaned and dissected and the removal of the entire prostate gland is generally begun at the end that is farthest from the bladder, next to the external urethral sphincter. The prostatic urethra is divided at this point; then it and the prostate gland through which it goes are pulled upward toward the bladder while the dissection continues behind the prostate gland separating it from the layer of tissue that is connected to the rectum on its other side. As the dissection continues between the prostate and the rectum, the seminal vesicles, which are behind the base of the bladder, come into view and are removed along with the prostate gland. This dissection of the seminal vesicles from the back wall of the bladder is generally done after the bladder neck has been cut across. Once the seminal vesicles are free, the entire prostate gland and the seminal vesicles are removed. The bladder neck is tailored to a small enough diameter so that it is about the same size as the stump of the urethra from which the prostate was detached. The bladder neck is then pulled down into the

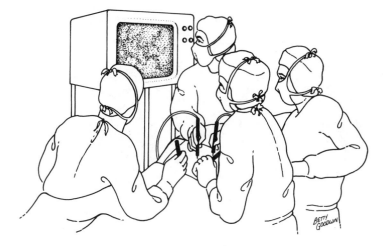

Figure 6–12   *Operating room setup for laparoscopic surgery. Note the four instruments protruding from the patient's abdominal cavity. Three of these are dissecting or grasping instruments, and the fourth is a camera with a light source that enables the members of the operating team to view on the TV screen what is being seen and done by the surgeon within the abdominal cavity.*

pelvis and snugged up against the urethral stump and stitched to it (Fig. 6–13). The stitching is done around a Foley catheter which has been inserted through the penis all the way into the bladder.

The entire operation is a formidable one, generally taking at least two hours and often taking more than three hours. There is not infrequently a considerable loss of blood. Recovery from surgery is usually slower than from any of the forms of surgery that are done for BPH. The patient is generally in the hospital for two to five days and is then sent home with a catheter in place. This catheter is left in place for about two weeks from the time of surgery and is removed on a postoperative visit. The reason the catheter is left in place is to permit the healing in the area where the bladder neck was stitched to the stump of the urethra and to minimize any leakage of urine through this stitched area.

The second alternative surgical approach that is used for a radical prostatectomy is through the perineum, the area

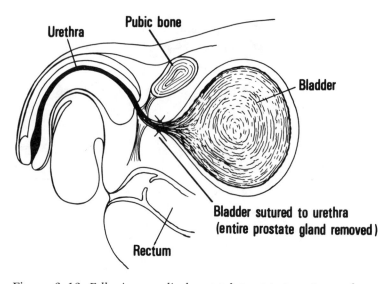

Figure 6–13 *Following a radical, or total, prostatectomy (removal of the prostate) by either the perineal or the retropubic approach, the bladder neck is sutured to the stump of the urethra. The entire prostate gland has been removed.*

between the scrotum and the anus. This approach is called a radical perineal prostatectomy. Some surgeons definitely prefer this approach, and there is no question that there is considerably less blood loss when this approach is used. As noted earlier, the only real disadvantage of this approach (other than the fact that most urologists are not comfortable with it because of a relative unfamiliarity with the anatomy of the area) is that it is not possible to sample the lymph nodes of the pelvis when this approach is used. As already noted, such sampling may not always be necessary and can be done laparoscopically if indicated. It should finally be noted that this perineal approach is easier on the patient in terms of postoperative discomfort and time to recovery.

The surgical incision that is used for a radical perineal prostatectomy is usually in the shape of an inverted U falling right over the anus, with the center of the U about 3 centimeters above the margin of the anus. In extending the incision deep into the tissues of the perineum, it is important to release the attachments of the rectum to the urethra so the rectum will fall away toward the back of the patient while the urethra and ultimately the prostate gland are more anterior, so the chance of damaging the rectum is minimized. The prostate gland is freed from its surrounding structures by gentle dissection and the urethra at the end of the prostate farthest from the bladder is isolated and divided. The bladder neck is freed from the prostate, and once the prostate gland has been removed and the bladder neck has been closed sufficiently so that the sides of its opening approximate the size of the urethral opening, the urethra and bladder neck are stitched together. As with the radical retropubic prostatectomy, a catheter is left in place postoperatively for two to three weeks.

Cryoablation of the Prostate

This is a procedure in which some urologists fervently believe; and it is used to treat cancer of the prostate in selected patients by freezing the cancer with liquid nitrogen. It is done with the patient either asleep or under spinal anesthesia. Several probes are placed, guided by ultrasound, through the patient's perineum (the area between the anus and the scrotum) into his prostate gland. Each of these probes is a little larger than 3 millimeters in diameter. Liquid nitrogen is then introduced through these probes into the prostate gland, and a little ice ball can be seen to form at the end of each probe as it is viewed on the ultrasound screen.

This procedure for the treatment of prostate cancer certainly has its adherents but I do believe they are getting fewer as time goes by. There is no question that this freezing procedure can destroy prostate cancer, but there is also a steep learning curve with this procedure and complications can be significant when it is undertaken. Both impotence and retrograde ejaculation can and do occur following this procedure, and although it still has many adherents and must be considered as a possible therapy for prostate cancer, I do believe that the vast majority of urologists consider cryoablation of the prostate a less than optimal method of treating prostate cancer when compared with radical prostatectomy or any of the forms of radiation therapy (external beam, implantation of radioactive seeds, or a combination of the two).

Laparoscopic Radical Prostatectomy

There are very few urologists at this point in time who are skilled enough to do a radical prostatectomy laparoscopically, and most of these procedures have been done in Western Europe. The number of them done annually in the United States is minuscule, although future years may find this procedure is the standard surgical treatment for prostate cancer. As of now, it is questionable if it significantly minimizes duration of hospital stay, expense, or patient morbidity.

Bilateral Orchiectomy (Removal of the Testes)

In the early 1940s it was conclusively demonstrated that the great majority (around 90 percent) of prostate cancers are dependent on the male hormone testosterone for growth. This means that the growth and spread of prostatic carcinoma (in 90 percent of patients) is enhanced by normal circulating blood levels of testosterone. More importantly, it means that the growth and spread of prostate carcinoma is markedly slowed by removal of the testosterone. It has long been known, because of this basic research on the influence of male hormones on the spread of prostate cancer, that prostate cancer patients live longer and with a better quality of life in the absence of any circulating testosterone. Although definitely not curative, the removal of testosterone has been proven to significantly palliate patients with prostate cancer that has spread outside the confines of the prostate gland. The patients for whom removal of testosterone may be considered beneficial are those patients in whom there is documented spread of cancer to the pelvic lymph nodes, to the bones, or anywhere else in the body. Removal of testosterone is *not* considered for any patients in whom the cancer is presumably confined to the prostate gland and therefore is potentially curable.

Although there are several ways to reduce the circulating testosterone to near zero levels (see Chapter 5), removal of the testes (bilateral orchiectomy) has been considered for many years to be the most efficient way. Unfortunately, this operation is one that is understandably dreaded and feared by most men; for this reason it is often refused in favor of another procedure, the injection of LH-RH hormones, which is every bit as successful as bilateral orchiectomy in retarding the course of the cancer but which may be prohibitively expensive. It is estimated that the administration of LH-RH agonist hormones, whether done monthly or at three- to four-month intervals, costs between $6,000 and $8,000 per year at a minimum.

Many patients for whom bilateral orchiectomy is recommended are beyond the point in life when sexual intercourse is important. Regardless, what seems to be anathema to most men about bilateral orchiectomy is almost unrelated to intercourse itself and strikes at the very core of maleness—emasculation in an intellectual sense. Certainly this is the problem for most men who are no longer really interested in sexual intercourse. Bilateral orchiectomy, in and of itself, does not necessarily lead to impotence, and there are indeed men who continue to get erections after the surgery. It does, however, lead to a loss of libido in most men, and this is true whether the hormone deprivation is by bilateral orchiectomy or by the administration of LH-RH agonist hormones. For those men who still want to pursue an active sex life, however, there are several very viable options (see Chapter 8).

The operation of bilateral orchiectomy is a very simple one that may be done under local or general anesthesia and usually does not involve an overnight stay in the hospital. A small incision, no more than 1 or 2 inches in length, is usually made in the middle portion of the lower part of the scrotum (between the two testes), and both testes can easily be removed through this one incision. Alternatively, some urologists like to make small incisions on each side of the scrotum through which the respective testes can be removed. The scrotum itself has relatively few pain fibers; so the postoperative course is marked by minimal discomfort, and the scrotal incision heals rapidly and well because of the normally excellent blood supply to the scrotum. Bilateral orchiectomy is such a relatively minor surgical procedure, in fact, that it is almost always done on an outpatient basis.

Unfortunately, some urologists, accustomed to caring for patients with prostatic carcinoma, become quite callous to the mental trauma inflicted on a patient who has to be told that his testes need to be removed. Not infrequently, an earthy form of language is used to tell the patient what needs to be done, and it is a rare man, indeed, who is not totally shattered by this news. Many urologists tend to be quite upset with patients who refuse the recommendation for this operation and who opt instead for the alternative form of injectable hormonal therapy. It has always been my policy to make a point of sitting down with my patient and trying to discuss the recommendation of bilateral orchiectomy in a very private setting and particularly in a very unhurried manner. I have found that many patients will ultimately go along with bilateral orchiectomy once they understand the shortcomings of the alternative therapy (the need to visit the doctor on a frequent and regular basis to receive the hormone injections as well as the very prohibitive cost which is, however, often borne by the insurance carrier) and once they realize that their own self-image and self-worth are not totally contained in their testes. For those patients, however, who adamantly refuse orchiectomy, I will always pursue the alternative means of treatment.

Radiation Therapy for Prostate Cancer

One of the time-honored, recognized, and widely used forms for therapy of prostate cancer is radiation therapy. My own bias in favor of surgical treatment reflects, in part, the fact that I am a surgeon; but I also like to think that it reflects my very genuine belief that there are more hard data showing that the cure rate and the long-term survival without any clinical evidence of residual cancer is significantly better with surgical treatment, particularly when the data extend beyond ten years from the time of treatment. Nevertheless, as better and better radiation therapy techniques become available, there is no question that radiation therapy is a very valid and fine means of treating prostate cancer. It is unquestionably preferred and chosen by and for many patients, and for this reason I believe a brief discussion of this treatment should be included. There are two different forms of radiation therapy currently being used in the United States, and sometimes these two are combined.

One is the form known as external beam radiation therapy. Most recently, with the availability of better radiation therapy equipment, better computers, and the most-sophisticated means of delivering this therapy, it is more possible than ever to conform the radiation therapy to the configuration of the prostate and thereby spare any harmful effects to the rectum and the bladder. This is known as *conformal* radiation therapy. It is given as external beam therapy usually in a dosage of 70 grays over a seven-week period. Many radiation therapists like to combine this with hormone deprivation therapy using LH-RH agonists for about three months prior to the external beam therapy to shrink the prostate and hopefully make the radiation therapy even more effective. It is certainly a fair statement to say that in the very best of series, the results appear to be comparable to those achieved with surgery (radical prostatectomy), but I truly believe that for younger patients (those under 65) radical prostatectomy is the treatment of choice simply because I just do not believe that the very long-term beneficial effects of radiation therapy can equal those of radical prostatectomy. Nevertheless, it must be noted that radiation therapy is an excellent form of treatment and one which many patients choose.

The other type of radiation therapy that now appears to be the favorite form of radiation therapy in many communities is the implantation of radioactive material directly into the prostate, called brachytherapy. This is done using iodine 125 or palladium 103 seeds. These seeds are permanently implanted under a spinal anesthetic at one sitting into the prostate gland using ultrasound (or sometimes fluoroscopy) to localize them. The dosage of radiation therapy implanted when seeds are used is 144 grays. Another type of seed implant is temporary in the sense that needles are placed into the prostate and left protruding from the perineum, and periodically over a two-day period radioactive iridium 192 is placed through those needles into the prostate gland. For these two days the patient must stay in bed after which time the needles are removed and the radiation therapy is complete. It is felt by some radiation therapists that this implantation of radioactive material over a two-day period may be better for patients who have a higher risk of the spread of the cancer outside the prostate gland (this means immediately outside the prostate and not as far as the pelvic lymph nodes). Many radiation therapists choose to combine the implantation of permanent seeds with external beam therapy, and for such protocol the external beam is delivered over a five-week period in a dosage of 45 grays followed by a radioactive seed implant in a dosage of 90 grays.

The use of radioactive seeds is relatively new, and it is only possible to say that the very best of series suggests that the data of cancer-free survival for up to ten years appear to be about the same as with radical prostatectomy. Whether this will continue to hold beyond ten years, as it has with radical prostatectomy, remains to be seen. It should also be noted that combining preradiation hormone deprivation (using LH-RH agonists) for about three months with radiation therapy (seed implants or external beam or a combination of the two) after that has gained rather extensive usage among some radiation therapists who have not been happy with the results of external beam therapy alone.

Within six to twelve months following the completion of whatever form of radiation therapy (external beam, seeds, or both) is used, the PSA should reach its nadir and this should be less than 1 nanogram per milliliter. Ideally, it should be less than 0.5 nanogram per milliliter. It will not usually go to undetectable levels (as it should after a radical prostatectomy) because the patient still has his prostate gland and that gland will usually still be making some PSA. However, if the PSA never gets below 1 nanogram per milliliter, this may mean that the radiation has not destroyed all the cancer cells. The patient is monitored with PSA blood tests, and if the PSA continues to rise, further treatment may be indicated. This could consist of hormonal therapy or of a "salvage" prostatectomy where the radiated prostate gland is removed. This procedure has a high (up to 50 percent) likelihood of postoperative incontinence. Another option is cryoablation which in this case may be the best option.

To sum up, radiation therapy has much to offer patients and should definitely be considered by any patient who is a candidate for curative treatment of prostatic carcinoma. I have always referred every single one of my patients who fall into this category to our radiation therapist for consultation, and after that the patient can decide whether he wants radiation therapy or a radical prostatectomy. In my own experience, about half of the patients opt for radiation and about half for surgery.

It should finally be noted that there is about a 2 percent incidence of severe complications following radiation therapy, including such things as incontinence, intractable bleeding from the bladder, and permanent damage to the rectum. There is about a 5 percent incidence of more transient and moderate complications involving the bladder and rectum as well. Overall, radiation therapy is a thoroughly acceptable and valid form of treatment for prostate cancer that is confined within the prostate gland (stages A, B, or C, or stages T1, T2, or T3), and the very best of the data regarding the results of radiation therapy suggests that it is possibly as efficacious as radical prostatectomy in the treatment of prostate cancer. However, I feel that these data are perhaps somewhat soft in that they do not provide the duration of follow-up or the very great numbers of patients that can be found in analyzing the results of radical prostatectomy in the treatment of patients with prostate cancer. Therefore, it is my very strong feeling that the younger the patient, the greater is the need for radical prostatectomy because a young patient presumably would have many more years of life absent the prostate cancer than an older patient would. I feel that a radical prostatectomy is preferable to radiation therapy (whether external beam or seeds or combined) for patients who are younger than 60 years of age and, usually, for patients who are younger than 70 years of age.

7

What You (the Patient) Can Anticipate at Each Step along the Way

If You Go to Your Doctor with Symptoms of Prostatic Inflammation or Infection or with the Chronic Pelvic Pain Syndrome

Probably the first, and perhaps the most important thing, that your doctor will do is to take a detailed medical history from you about your present symptoms, your past genitourinary tract symptoms or problems, and your health in general. All of this is very important in helping your doctor reach a correct diagnosis, and you should search your memory carefully and be honest about the answers you provide.

You will certainly be asked what specific problem or complaint brought you to the doctor. The answer to this is what physicians call the "chief complaint." Was it pain in the area between your scrotum and anus (the perineum)? Was it pain in your rectum? Was it pain or discomfort deep inside your penis? Was it pain with ejaculation? Have you had any sort of abnormal or unusual discharge from the penis? Have you had any burning or other discomfort during urination? Has your urine had a foul odor? Have you had fever accompanying your symptoms? Have you had pain anywhere else along with your symptoms? For how long have your present symptoms been bothering you? Have you ever been definitely diagnosed with a urinary tract infection? Have you ever before had any symptoms like the present ones? If so, how were you treated? Have you ever seen a urologist before for any of your present

symptoms or similar ones? Have you ever had *any* other urologic complaints? Blood in your urine? Kidney stones? Any
childhood history of urologic symptoms or disease? Your doctor may also give you a very new form to fill out that is known
as the NIH-Chronic Prostatitis Symptom Index. This is a val-
idated symptom evaluation tool that can be used in helping
your physician to understand and to treat your problem.

Your physician will then ask you many questions pertaining to your sex life and your sexual history. This is extremely
important so you should make every effort to be as honest and
straightforward with your answers as possible. The reason
your physician does this is because it is very common for men
to come to a physician (particularly to a urologist) complaining of a genitourinary problem or symptom when the *real* reason the patient has come to the physician is because of a sexual
problem. Most patients are reluctant to talk about their sexual problems, real or imagined. The astute physician realizes
this and will ask questions during the course of the medical
history to determine if indeed there is a sexual problem. You
will be asked questions such as: Do you have any difficulty
achieving erections? Are the erections sufficient for vaginal
penetration? Are you able to keep your erections long enough
to allow for vaginal penetration and orgasm? Is there anything
at all about your sexual life that you would care to discuss?

Your physician will next ask you questions about your
health in general, questions that are important for their own
sake but could also impact on your specific urologic problem.
Do you have diabetes or is there any family history of diabetes? Do you have high blood pressure, are you being treated for high blood pressure, or have you ever been treated for
high blood pressure? Have you ever been told that you have
tuberculosis or is there any history in your family of tuberculosis? Are you allergic to any medications? Are you allergic to
anything of which you are aware, and if so, what?

Your physician will next perform a physical examination,
and the extent of the examination will depend in large measure on whether your physician is a primary care physician or
a urologist. If the former, he will probably do a reasonably
complete, albeit cursory, examination. If he is a urologist, he
will probably confine his examination to the genitourinary
tract which is, after all, that part of the body related to the reason that you have come to see him. You will probably start the

examination by lying flat on your back on an examining table while the doctor quickly palpates your abdomen. This is simply to look for any lumps, bumps, or areas of pain or tenderness, or even an enlargement of your bladder which might suggest incomplete bladder emptying. He will next examine your genitals, usually while you are still lying on your back. This is important because it will enable your physician to determine the normalcy of your penis and testes. Remember that cancer of the testes is the most common form of solid cancer in males between the ages of 18 and 40, and it usually produces no symptoms at all. It is diagnosed only by a physical examination or by the patient doing a self-examination. Your physician will next ask you to stand up, at which time he will check you for a hernia in your groin area and for any abnormalities that might exist in your scrotum.

Now, considering the fact that you have come to the physician because of a set of symptoms that suggest you may have inflammation or infection in your prostate gland or in your prostatic urethra (see Chapter 3), it is absolutely necessary that your physician determine with certainty if it is your prostate or your urethra that is the source of your difficulty. If it is your prostate, is it inflammation in that gland or is it infection? These questions are answered by a laboratory test of your urine. To do this, your doctor will ask you to start to void into a sterile container that is marked #1. You will do this, putting perhaps an ounce or two of urine into the glass, and then, without stopping your urinary stream, you will direct it out of glass #1 and briefly into the toilet before directing it into an empty sterile container marked #2. After voiding a couple of ounces of urine into the second glass, which will be the midstream urine, you will move glass #2 away from your urinary stream (without stopping your stream) and void directly into the toilet, being certain to retain some urine in your bladder for what is to follow.

Your physician will then do a digital rectal examination of your prostate and will "strip," or "massage," your prostate vigorously (see Chapter 3) so as to express secretions from the prostate gland into the prostatic urethra. During this time, you will grasp the end of your penis and keep it squeezed tightly shut so that none of the prostatic secretions escape during this prostatic massage. This prostatic stripping, or massage, is certainly not pleasant, but neither is it painful and most patients feel that its worst aspect is the forceful feeling that some fluid (the prostatic fluid) is trying to come out of the urethra. In point of fact, there is often no fluid that comes out of the urethra at the conclusion of the prostatic massage; but if any does appear, it is collected for microscopic examination and culture. Most of the time the prostatic secretions have just pooled in the prostatic urethra, and to obtain them for examination, you will be asked to void one more time into a glass marked #3. Into this container you will put an ounce or two of urine, which will then contain the secretions from the prostate gland. At this point, you will simply finish emptying your bladder into the toilet.

It is the comparison between the number of bacteria in the three glasses of urine as well as the microscopic appearance of the prostatic secretions themselves (if any have been obtained) that will enable your doctor to tell you whether your symptoms are due to infection or inflammation in the prostate gland or infection in the urethra (or neither). If your doctor determines that your problem is in your urethra or your prostate, she will be able to treat you. If the infection is in the prostatic portion of the urethra, where it will almost always be when there is a urethral infection (except for gonorrheal infection), the drug of choice is tetracycline or one of its synthetic derivatives; therapy is usually continued for two or three weeks. If you have infection in your prostate gland (and this is very uncommon), the treatment will usually be with Bactrim or Septra (they are the same drug made by two different companies), or one of the fluoroquinolones such as ciprofloxacin (Cipro) or levofloxacin (Levaquin), depending on the bacteria identified in the prostatic secretions. Treatment is usually necessary for at least a month and often for up to three months; but the treatment of chronic bacterial infection in the prostate is by no means always successful, and probably no more than one-half to two-thirds of patients with chronic bacterial infection achieve an eradication of the infection. The remaining patients may well have recurring infections over a period of many years.

If you have a simple inflammation without any bacterial infection in your prostate, your doctor may give you an antibiotic for one or two weeks, and you will be absolutely delighted when your physician additionally prescribes for you a program of frequent intercourse or masturbation since some physicians feel that inflammation of the prostate gland may result from inadequate, infrequent, or incomplete emptying of the prostate gland, something that may be caused by a sudden diminution in the frequency of ejaculation. The treatment of this condition is therefore a singularly joyous one that most men appreciate greatly. Many patients have achieved relief from a nonbacterial inflammation in the prostate gland by repeated courses of vigorous prostatic massage combined with antibiotics, and the rationale for this is to forcibly strip, or empty, the prostate of these inflammatory cells and perhaps any bacteria that may be present.

It is worthwhile noting, however, that the information on nonbacterial inflammation within the prostate gland is very soft. When large numbers of men have prostate biopsies (which are done for reasons unrelated to prostatic inflammation or infection), over half of these biopsies show pathologic evidence of chronic inflammation of the prostate; yet most of these men do not have and never have had any symptoms that would suggest prostatic inflammation. It is certainly possible that prostatic inflammation may be due to organisms within the prostate that have thus far avoided any detection and that future research may reveal such organisms. I am personally not very sanguine that this is the situation, however. In the absence of any definite evidence of bacterial infection in the prostate (see Chapter 3), it may be very difficult or even impossible to say that a man's prostate gland is the source of his discomfort. Conditions such as interstitial cystitis, bladder tumor, inflammation and spasm of the muscles of the floor of the perineum, an imbalance between bladder contraction and relaxation of the urethral sphincter, spinal problems, and others are all conditions that can simulate the extremely variable symptoms men commonly associate with prostatitis.

When one of my patients has such symptoms (as noted at the beginning of this chapter) and I can find no evidence of any bacterial infection, I recommend a cystoscopic examination to see if there is any suggestion of interstitial cystitis and also to be sure no tumor is present. I will perform a urodynamic study to see if there are any abnormalities in the physiology of my patient's voiding pattern. Sometimes a magnetic resonance study of the lower back will reveal spinal abnormalities that can account for the patient's symptoms. Treatment of such problems can indeed be difficult and can encompass such things as biofeedback, smooth muscle relaxant medications such as Valium, medications such as amitriptyline which often has a salutary effect on such problems, and sometimes even an alpha blocker such as Hytrin or Cardura may help. The indeterminate nature of the cause of these symptoms and the desire not to focus a man's disability on what is often an innocent prostate gland are the reasons that these varied symptoms are perferably referred to as chronic pelvic pain syndrome.

Some physicians tell patients who have any or many of these symptoms that they should abstain from alcohol or any spicy or hot foods. The rationale for this is that these things, absorbed from the stomach into the bloodstream, may eventually reach the urine in concentrations high enough to cause the patient discomfort when the urine passes over the presumably inflamed lining of the prostatic urethra. I do not agree at all with this thesis, and I tell my patients that it is perfectly all right for them to eat or drink anything they want; they will do no harm whatever to their prostate gland or their prostatic urethra. However, I also tell my patients that if alcohol or any spicy or hot foods *do* cause them discomfort when they are urinating, they might want to consider no longer drinking or eating them. It is up to the patient to make this decision.

If You Go to Your Doctor with Symptoms of Benign Prostatic Hyperplasia (BPH)

You will probably go to see your doctor because you are getting up too many times at night to urinate or you are urinating too frequently or you feel you are not emptying your bladder or you are wetting your pants after you think you have finished voiding. In any case, your doctor certainly will ask you many questions to confirm his very preliminary impression that you have BPH. The chances are that he would have this impression only on the basis of your presenting complaint and the fact that you are over 45 years of age. The older you are when you first see your physician with these complaints, the more likely he will be to think that your diagnosis is BPH.

Nevertheless, undoubtedly your physician will ask you

many questions, all of which are designed to confirm his initial impression that BPH is your problem. How many times do you get up at night? Do you have trouble starting your urinary stream? Does your urinary stream ever stop completely before your finish voiding and then start up again some seconds later? Do you feel as if you empty your bladder when you void? Is your urinary stream noticeably weaker than it was five years ago? Have you ever had any pain or discomfort of burning while urinating? When you get the urge to urinate do you have to do it right away or can you wait until a convenient time presents itself? Have you ever lost any urine involuntarily? Have you ever seen any blood in your urine? All of these questions will help your doctor to diagnose BPH since any or all of these symptoms are associated with this condition.

There are, however, other conditions which will enter your physician's mind when he listens to your litany of symptoms. Some of the conditions which must be differentiated from BPH primarily involve abnormalities of your bladder that may be completely unrelated to your prostate, and these fall into two general categories. A hyperactive or an overactive bladder can lead to the symptoms of frequency, urgency, nocturia, and even urge incontinence. An atonic, or flabby, bladder cannot generate enough pressure to void with a good and normal stream and can lead to the symptoms of difficulty starting the stream, intermittency, a very weak urinary stream, and a feeling of incomplete bladder emptying. Both of these bladder problems *can* be caused by an obstructing prostate gland but they can *also* be primary bladder problems unrelated to any prostatic obstruction. It therefore is the prudent physician who suggests a pressure/flow study to differentiate a primary bladder problem from a problem that is caused because of a bladder outlet obstruction due to BPH (see Chapter 2 and Chapter 4 for details about these pressure/flow studies and how they are done).

Scarring or stricture in the urethra can also lead to the symptoms commonly associated with BPH and can be due to an old gonorrheal infection or to some sort of injury that was done to the urethra in the past such as by the presence of a Foley catheter for more than a brief period of time or even a cystoscopy that was done when the patient was a child. Such urethral scarring or stricture can usually be diagnosed by a careful history regarding when the patient's symptoms began.

If the patient has not had any symptoms of voiding difficulty until the relatively recent past and nothing has transpired lately that could have led to a urethral stricture or scar, then that possible diagnosis is obviously not a tenable one. Similarly, a bladder neck contraction, unless it has followed a previous operation on the prostate, would have been present since a very early age and the history of voiding difficulty would go back for many years.

The physical examination starts with the abdomen, and a particular emphasis is placed on looking for an enlarged or distended bladder since this finding may go along with BPH. The digital rectal examination helps to estimate the size of the prostate gland, and therefore the BPH enlargement. It also is done to be sure there are no hard or firm areas in the prostate that might be suggestive of malignancy. What your doctor is *not* able to do on a digital rectal examination of the prostate is to state unequivocally that you do or do not have BPH that is responsible for your symptoms. This is because a normal-sized prostate can still result in profound obstruction to the flow of urine. The obstruction would be due to an enlarged middle lobe of the prostate which cannot be palpated on digital rectal examination but which in fact is the most common cause of the symptoms of BPH. Also, even if the prostate gland were noticeably enlarged, this would only be suggestive and not confirmative of lateral lobe enlargement that is encroaching on the prostatic urethra and hindering the flow of urine (see Chapter 4 for a detailed discussion of BPH).

While your physician is doing the digital rectal examination, he will often perform a bulbocavernosus reflex test by briskly squeezing the head of your penis while his finger is in your rectum. The absence of a contraction of the anal sphincter on his finger that is in your rectum would suggest that there might be an abnormality in your bladder innervation and this, as already noted, can be ruled in or ruled out with a pressure/flow study.

A urinalysis is usually done at this point, primarily to look for white blood cells (pus cells) which might indicate the presence of infection in the urine. If white cells are present, the urine should be cultured. If there is any suggestion of past or present history of urinary tract infection, the urine should also be cultured.

Blood is obtained from a vein in your arm for creatinine

and blood urea nitrogen tests (see Chapter 2) in order to evaluate your kidney function. A blood prostate specific antigen test is done as well, and if the PSA level is elevated, it may indicate that you should have a biopsy of your prostate gland because of the possibility of prostate cancer (see Chapter 2). The presence of prostate cancer would in some cases have been suggested by an abnormal digital rectal examination; however, in the great majority of patients in whom prostate cancer is diagnosed nowadays, the rectal examination will suggest an entirely benign gland and it is only the elevated PSA blood test level that leads to the prostate biopsy which in turn leads to the diagnosis of prostate cancer.

You may recall from Chapter 4 that there are two broad sets of indications, subjective and objective, for treatment to relieve the symptoms of benign prostatic hyperplasia. First (subjective), treatment may be indicated when a patient's findings of bladder outlet obstruction are bothersome enough that he would like relief from them, and second (objective), treatment is probably necessary when there is definite objective evidence of an inability to empty the bladder, back pressure on the kidneys, deteriorating kidney function, recurrent urinary tract infections, or more than one episode of acute urinary retention. To evaluate this second broad category of indications for treatment (the objective category), your doctor may perform several studies, including an evaluation of your kidneys to see if there is any significant back pressure on them due to incomplete bladder emptying.

This determination is usually done with an imaging study and it may be either an ultrasound examination or an excretory urogram that would be done (see Chapter 2). If your doctor does one of these studies to see if there is back pressure on your kidneys, she will probably also want to evaluate your bladder for the presence or absence of residual urine following voiding, and this is commonly done with a bladder ultrasound examination. If you tell your doctor that you have moderate symptoms of voiding difficulty and your real concern is whether you need to have any treatment for this, your doctor will realize that your symptoms alone may not warrant any treatment but she will also realize that it is important to be certain that you are not slowly damaging your kidneys because of back pressure on them from an incompletely emptied bladder. A bladder ultrasound and an ultrasound examination of your kidneys will show if there is any such back pressure, and it will also show how well you empty your bladder. On the basis of the history you have given to your physician, a physical examination, perhaps a pressure/flow study, and any imaging studies that may have been done, your doctor now feels that it is quite likely that you do indeed have obstruction to your flow of urine from an enlargement of your prostate gland. At this point, your physician may possibly want to cystoscope you (see Chapter 2) because this will permit an actual look at the existing obstruction to the flow of urine. It is important that you should realize that this cystoscopic examination cannot tell your physician anything about whether your prostate is obstructing your bladder but it can give your urologist information about the anatomic configuration of your prostate gland. So your physician may well want to do a cystoscopic examination if she feels that prostate surgery is indicated and she is trying to determine after looking at the prostatic urethra what type of surgical procedure she should recommend to you.

If you do have a cystoscopic examination, note that this can be done with either a rigid cystoscope or a flexible cystoscope (see Fig. 2–10). If it is done with a rigid cystoscope, you will be placed in the lithotomy position, and if a flexible cystoscope is used, you will be placed flat on your back on the cystoscopy table. Regardless of the instrument used, the urethra is well anesthetized using an anesthetic jelly squirted into it and then the instrument is introduced into the urethral opening at the tip of your penis and very slowly and gently advanced up through the penile urethra and the prostatic urethra and finally into the bladder. When it is in the prostatic urethra, and the light and lens are about at the level of the external urethral sphincter, the physician can estimate the amount and the configuration of obstructing prostatic tissue. I must emphasize again, however, that the only thing your urologist will be able to see is the extent of *anatomic* obstruction. The cystoscopic exam is unable to reveal anything about the *functional* obstruction. In other words, I believe that the cystoscopic exam is not really very helpful in determining whether a patient should have prostate surgery; rather, once the decision has been made that a surgical intervention is necessary, a cystoscopy may help to determine which specific surgical approach would be optimal. Whether this cystoscopic examination is done in the office or at the time of the surgical intervention to treat the patient is really an individual choice of the given urologist. The other reason for doing a cystoscopic examination is to be sure that no coexisting pathology within the bladder (such as cancer) exists.

The cystoscopic examination, when it is done as an office procedure, could not be called pleasant or totally without discomfort; but it certainly is not a painful exam as long as local anesthetic is used and the urologist is gentle and skilled.

For a cystoscopic exam in the doctor's office, if a rigid instrument is used, you will be placed on an examining table with your legs spread wide apart and supports placed behind your knees to hold them in an elevated position. This is known as the lithotomy position and is very similar to the position in which a woman is placed when she is about to give birth. Your genitals will be washed with soap and water and perhaps with a disinfectant or antiseptic solution. A local anesthetic, usually in jelly form, will then be squirted into your urethra, and ideally it is supposed to go all the way down the urethra and into the bladder. The local anesthetic that I use is a jelly that comes out of a tube that looks very much like a toothpaste tube, and the little nozzle at the end of the tube is inserted into the opening at the end of the penis. The tube itself is then briskly squeezed, so the jelly is forced into the urethra. To some patients, this is the most unpleasant part of the entire procedure.

After allowing five to ten minutes for the anesthetic to work, the cystoscope is introduced into the urethra and very gently advanced into the bladder. When the instrument is in place, you should not feel any pain but you will be aware of the sensation that something is inside you. Your urologist will probably take between two and five minutes for the entire procedure and may use two different lenses to examine you; one of these is optimal for the bladder examination and one for the examination of the prostatic urethra. I have not found it necessary to use any injectable tranquilizers or pain killers to facilitate cystoscopy, although some urologists do use these. My concern is simply that when such medications are used, it is generally not safe for the patient to drive his car for several hours. Note that all of the foregoing pertains equally to the cystoscopic procedure that is done with a flexible instrument except that you will be flat on your back when the flexible instrument is used and only one lens is used when the flexible instrument is employed.

When all of the above studies or as many of them as the urologist feels are indicated have been finished and the evidence points to the need for prostate surgery, the question invariably comes up, "How soon?" There is usually a good bit of leeway here and you should frankly discuss your desires and feelings with your physician. If the indications for surgery consist only of the symptoms that you have when you void, I feel that you as the patient should make the decision as to when you want the surgery. It is my practice never to push or urge a patient to have surgery sooner than he desires as long as the indications for surgery are limited to the patient's own voiding problems.

I believe that medical treatment (see Chapter 4) is worth trying in most patients who have only the subjective indications for surgery because this treatment will, in my experience, benefit at least half of the patients trying it. However, there are some patients who do not want to take pills every day or who cannot otherwise tolerate these medications, and in such patients surgery is indeed indicated.

As noted before, other patients will have objective findings that I feel make the timing of surgery perhaps a bit less flexible than when only subjective symptoms are present. These objective findings are those which, if not reversed, can well lead to kidney damage, recurring infection, and inability to void or even uremic poisoning. Once the postvoid residual urine gets much over 100–150 cubic centimeters, I believe that surgery should be seriously considered. Medical therapy can always be tried but I have not found it to be very beneficial in such patients. Once a patient has had one episode of bladder infection, I feel that he will inevitably get future infections unless the residual urine that predisposed him to infection is eliminated. Once there is evidence of back pressure on the kidneys, I believe that treatment to relieve such back pressure should be done sooner rather than later. Certainly prostate surgery in any case is never the emergency that it might be with, say, acute appendicitis; but a general rule of thumb is that when there are objective indications for prostate surgery, it should be done at a relatively early time and one that is best suited for both the patient and the physician.

Once the decision has been made to proceed with prostate

surgery for the relief of BPH, you will often feel a sense of relief because you have made the decision to go ahead and you know that your bothersome symptoms of prostate disease will hopefully be a thing of the past. The results of surgery for prostatic obstruction are quite excellent if you do truly have prostatic obstruction as determined by the pressure/flow study.

If you are going to have one of the minimally invasive procedures to relieve your bladder outlet obstruction, it can often be done right in your physician's office. These procedures are the microwave thermotherapy and the TransUrethral Needle Ablation of the prostate (TUNA). For one of the relatively more invasive procedures (such as a laser treatment of your prostate, a vaporization procedure, a TUIP, a TURP, or even an open operation on your prostate), you will be admitted to the hospital or, in some cases, to the same-day unit of the hospital and you will have a general physical examination to assess your overall condition (see Chapter 6). This is usually done by your family physician or internist, but it may also be done by a resident physician or by your urologist. You may have a chest x-ray and an electrocardiogram as well as basic laboratory work and urine tests prior to surgery. This will depend on the procedure you are having done and whether it is being done in an office, a same-day unit, or an inpatient unit in the hospital. If you are to have any sort of spinal or general anesthesia, an anesthesiologist will most likely visit with you to discuss your choice of anesthesia, and you should share with the anesthesiologist your preferences and any fears or concerns you may have.

For patients having a TUNA procedure or a microwave thermotherapy procedure, no anesthesia is usually necessary other than perhaps some intraurethral medication or sometimes a prostate block or some intravenous sedation (for the TUNA). For almost all of the other prostate operative procedures, a spinal anesthesia is preferred over a general anesthetic and the reasons for this are twofold. First, the muscles of the lower abdomen and pelvic floor are usually more relaxed with a spinal anesthetic; second, there are none of the lung complications with a spinal anesthetic that sometimes are present after a general or inhalational anesthetic. With a general anesthetic some patients develop a collapse of small segments of the lung; other patients develop a pneumonia in some portions of the lung. Although these are invariably treated successfully, the fact remains that with spinal anesthesia these complications virtually never occur. There are certain reasons the anesthesiologist may have for *not* wanting to perform spinal anesthesia. Two of these are previous spinal surgery or spinal injury and certain types of cardiovascular disease that do not tolerate drops in blood pressure which frequently accompany spinal anesthesia.

After one of the minimally invasive forms of treatment, you can usually go right home. You should have virtually no discomfort during the microwave thermotherapy ("heat" treatment) procedure, which will last between one and two hours. After it is finished, you will get up off the table and walk out, usually with an indwelling catheter for a couple of days. If you are having the TUNA procedure, there may be some discomfort during the procedure if the prostate block that was used for anesthesia is less than effective. This may need to be supplemented with some intravenous sedation but usually there is minimal discomfort during this procedure. You will also most likely need a catheter for a day or two.

If you are having one of the true surgical procedures to treat your prostatic enlargement, you will have a spinal anesthetic or perhaps a general anesthetic and you will not be at all uncomfortable regardless of the procedure or the approach that is taken. You will feel absolutely nothing if you have had a spinal anesthetic, and you will of course be asleep and therefore feel absolutely nothing if you are given a general or inhalational anesthetic. The operation itself will take anywhere from thirty minutes to two hours, and when it is finished, you will be in the recovery room, a special area where patients can be watched extraordinarily closely by highly trained nursing personnel as well as anesthesiologists, while they recover from the effects of the anesthesia and while they are in the immediate postoperative period. If your prostate surgery has been done via the transurethral route, you will have a catheter in your bladder following surgery. This would be the case whether you had a laser treatment, a vaporization treatment, a conventional TUIP, or a TURP. This catheter is placed through the penis and into the bladder, and it stays in place because of an inflatable bag that is larger than the size of the bladder neck (see Fig. 2–9) thereby preventing it from slipping out of the bladder.

If you have had a laser treatment or a vaporization of your prostate, you will have a catheter in your bladder for a couple of days and you may have continuous irrigation of your bladder through that catheter. There is usually a certain amount of bleeding from the part of the prostatic urethra where the surgery was done. This is minimal with a vaporization or a laser treatment of the prostate, but it may be more noticeable if you have had a conventional TURP or a TUIP. Usually, by the day after surgery or sometime the following day, it is possible to discontinue any continuous bladder irrigation and it is often possible to remove the catheter entirely. I generally remove the catheter on the day following surgery and sometimes it is possible to remove it the evening of surgery.

Following any of the endoscopic (through the penis) operative procedures on the prostate, you will have virtually no discomfort and certainly no pain following the procedure although there may occasionally be some bladder spasms which are usually due to the pressure of the inflatable catheter bag touching the very sensitive bladder trigone. These spasms can almost always be relieved or prevented by rectal suppositories of belladonna and opium which act directly on the bladder to relax it. It is very uncommon for a patient to require any narcotics postoperatively, and by the evening of the surgery you will most likely be eating and drinking food and fluids as desired and walking around your room or in the corridors of the hospital until you are discharged. The intravenous tubings that will be attached to you during surgery and immediately afterward are usually disconnected shortly after surgery once you have begun to drink fluids.

If you have had your prostate surgery done by one of the open approaches (the suprapubic or retropubic approach, see Chapter 6), you will undoubtedly have considerable pain and discomfort when your anesthesia (either spinal or general) wears off because the incision in your abdomen will be painful. The pain will be helped greatly by injections of whatever narcotic your doctor has prescribed; but you must remember that many nurses will not give you any narcotic for pain unless you specifically request it. In many hospitals a much-preferred method of delivering narcotic relief for pain in postoperative patients is now in place. This is referred to as Patient Controlled Analgesia. It consists of a machine that automatically monitors whatever narcotic is placed into it (usually morphine); so whenever you push a button that is by your bedside, a small dose of the narcotic leaves the machine and goes into the tubing that is providing you with your intravenous fluids. A lock-out mechanism prevents you from overdosing yourself with the narcotic and the amount that you receive with each push of the button combined with the fact that you are able to receive the narcotic virtually whenever you want it leads to a smooth and relatively pain-free postoperative period.

With the older but still in use method of the patient's having to ring for the nurse in order to get a narcotic shot, it is rather more the rule than the exception that the bell will not be answered promptly and, even if it is, the narcotic will not be delivered promptly. Consequently, the patient's pain gets to a nearly intolerable point by the time the injection is given. It is very interesting to note that in hospitals that have switched to the Patient Controlled Analgesia (PCA) machines, the total dose of narcotic received by each patient is actually less than the total narcotic dose that is received when it is given in isolated injections by the floor nurses.

If you have had a suprapubic approach to your prostate, you will have a tube coming out of your lower abdomen that goes straight into your bladder. This is in addition to the bladder catheter that is in your penis. If you have had a retropubic approach, you will have only one bladder catheter and that will be the one in your penis. The abdominal incisions and the pain from them are the same with either the suprapubic or the retropubic routes. When open surgery has been done, the catheters (either one or both) are allowed to drain freely to gravity drainage rather than with continuous irrigation. This is because during an open operation either the bladder or the true prostate capsule has been opened; if continuous irrigation were used and the outflow catheter should accidentally become plugged with a clot, the bladder or the true capsule of the prostate might be forcibly reopened by the resulting large collection of fluid in the bladder. With either of the open operations, you will probably require narcotics for several days postoperatively and will be in the hospital for anywhere from three to seven days following surgery. Some patients begin to drink fluids and to eat a soft diet the day after surgery, but most patients who have an open type of prostatectomy are really not eating very much until the third or fourth day following surgery.

Many men are seriously concerned about the consequences, emotional or physical, of moving their bowels on a daily basis. Following prostate surgery, your urologist will not want you to move your bowels for three or four days, at least, and this is especially true if your stools have a tendency to be particularly firm. This is because there is only a thin bit of connecting tissue between the rectum and the true capsule and true prostate tissue that normally remains behind after an operation for BPH. The pressure of a very large stool pressing against the true prostate gland so near the area from which the BPH was removed could stir up a considerable amount of bleeding from the site of the surgery. For the same reason it is extremely important that patients, during their hospital convalescence and for at least three weeks afterward, absolutely not strain at stool; this is best accomplished if a stool softener such as Metamucil is used.

The great majority of patients who have prostate surgery have uninfected urine prior to surgery. Nevertheless there are many physicians who feel more comfortable putting their patients on prophylactic antibiotics a day or two before surgery and continuing this through the hospitalization and for anywhere from two to six weeks postoperatively. It is my practice, however, not to use antibiotics unless there is a preoperative infection or unless the patient is in a high-risk group for infections, such as a diabetic or one who is on steroids. Should an infection occur during the convalescence, then antibiotics are of course used. But recall from an earlier chapter that the many white blood cells present in the urine during the first two or three months following surgery are *not* necessarily an indication of infection but only of the normal healing process that follows prostate surgery.

Any major surgical procedure, including true prostate surgery (not including the minimally invasive procedures), takes a lot more out of a patient than he may realize. You will find that it takes about one to three months following surgery before you will begin to feel like your old self again in terms of vigor, vitality, and a "get up and go" feeling. A lot of this will depend, of course, on your age; a younger man having the surgery will bounce back in just a few weeks. During this convalescence you should realize that the prostatic urethra, where the surgery was done, will not be totally healed with a new lining for about three months following surgery; and if you have an open operation, the muscles of your abdominal wall are not healed firmly for about six weeks postoperatively. Therefore, for at least six weeks after any kind of open prostate surgery, you should avoid intense physical exercise that could cause a disruption of the abdominal wound before all of the layers are firmly healed. For a similar length of time, you would be well advised to avoid any vigorous exercise and particularly any straining, lifting, or heavy work that could possibly result in bleeding from the site of the prostatic surgery. After about six weeks, even though the area of the surgical procedure has not yet healed completely, the risk of bleeding or any other complication is very minimal and patients are generally free to do whatever they choose, including a resumption of any sexual activities. I do, however, strongly advise my patients who have had any sort of prostate surgery not to do any sort of housework for a minimum of five years!

Up until the time the inside of the prostate gland is completely healed with its new lining, it certainly is possible that you may have some voiding discomfort and perhaps some frequency or urgency; you will probably have some nocturia as well. However, you will undoubtedly notice that your urinary stream is a strong one and it should be just about as large in caliber as your stream used to be when you were 20 years old! If you have a lot of frequency, though, you will be voiding often and in relatively small amounts, and so you may not always notice the good caliber and strength of your stream. When your bladder is full (at least 200 milliliters), you will indeed realize the formidable size and force of your urinary stream. As the area inside your prostate gland heals, any frequency, urgency, or burning on urination will gradually subside, although the nocturia may persist indefinitely. Getting up once or twice per night may well be nothing more than a residual habit from the years that you did this prior to your surgery, and this habit may remain forever. It does *not* mean that your surgery was unsuccessful.

I usually have my postoperative patients return to the office for follow-up care about two weeks after leaving the hospital, four to six weeks after that, and then again about six months postoperatively. These visits are made so the patient's progress in a normal and satisfactory manner can be verified and also to check the patient's urine to make sure there is no infection in it. I further recommend to my patients that they return annually thereafter. This is primarily so I can do a digital rectal exam of the prostate, as well as a blood prostate specific antigen (PSA) test, to try to detect any possible early findings suggestive of prostate cancer because, as will be remembered, the operation for BPH leaves behind the true prostate tissue which is the tissue in which prostate cancer originates.

A return to normal sexual activity is usually a relatively high priority for most patients; this should probably be deferred until the operative site is entirely healed, although it is not necessary to wait until the prostatic urethra has an entirely new lining. Within four to six weeks of surgery it is safe to resume full and normal sexual activity. Probably the only reason for not doing this any earlier is that the spasmodic contractions that occur in the prostatic urethra at the time of ejaculation could trigger delayed bleeding. Once six weeks or so following surgery have passed, the risk of a delayed bleed is very slight. From this time until the prostatic urethra is completely relined with normal mucosa, the only "risk" of intercourse is that there may be some discomfort at the time of ejaculation because the area going into spasm has not yet healed completely. As a general rule, those patients who achieved normal and full erections preoperatively can anticipate the return of these erections postoperatively any time after the catheter has been removed or within the first two to three weeks following surgery.

If Your Doctor Finds That You Have Prostatic Cancer

There can't be many words in the human language that are as fearsome as *cancer*. If your doctor should find it necessary to tell you that you have cancer in your prostate gland, it is particularly fearsome because you are absolutely certain that you will be impotent before long, and you will never again enjoy sexual intercourse. When your physician first suspects prostate cancer, the chances are good that you did not go to see him because of any urinary tract complaints but only for a routine physical examination. Alternatively, you may have gone to your physician for some totally unrelated problem such as a pain in your elbow or your shoulder, and when your physician takes the opportunity to do a thorough physical exam, he finds to his surprise and to your horror that there is a suspicious firm area that he has palpated on your prostate while doing a digital rectal examination. You will undoubtedly be referred to a urologist who will surely repeat the digital rectal examination in order to form an independent opinion about the suspicious area on your prostate. The urologist may then order a blood test consisting of a prostate specific antigen. Another scenario that is perhaps more common than the one just given is that your own physician, as part of a routine and general examination, has ordered a blood prostatic specific antigen test and the result has come back at an elevated level. Even though the digital rectal examination of your prostate was perfectly normal, your primary physician wisely refers you to a urologist.

With either of the above two scenarios, the urologist will undoubtedly feel that a prostatic biopsy is indicated, and this may be done in the urologist's office or in the hospital. Almost always these biopsies are done under ultrasound control, and if your urologist has such equipment in the office, the biopsy will undoubtedly be done there; otherwise it will be done in the radiology department of the hospital. The biopsy is done through the rectum (see Chapter 2), and it is not at all painful since the action of the biopsy "gun" is so rapid that the biopsy itself is virtually painless. Since the biopsy is performed through the rectum, cleansing laxatives are taken the night before and antibiotics are also used to minimize the chances of putting fecal bacteria into the prostate gland. Your urologist will undoubtedly use an ultrasound probe to first examine your prostate and then to guide the biopsy needle into the suspicious part of your prostate as well as into random other areas of your prostate gland. The ultrasound probe that is used for prostate examinations is about as big around as your thumb and it is inserted into your rectum for a distance of 3 to 4 inches when you are in a lying down position, usually on your side. It is not painful to insert this probe although it is certainly uncomfortable. Most urologists take at least six biopsies of the prostate, three from each lateral lobe, but more recent evidence has suggested that nine or even twelve biopsies should be done as this greatly increases the chances of finding any cancer that may be in the prostate.

If your biopsy suggests that you do indeed have prostate

cancer, your physician will notify you and request that you return to her or his office for discussions as to what should be done next. Obviously, it is important to determine if the prostate cancer is still confined within the prostate gland or if it has spread outside the gland. The best parameter that we urologists have for determining this is really the blood PSA level, and the lower it is, the less likelihood that the cancer has spread outside the prostate. As a matter of fact, if the PSA level is less than 10, most urologists do not recommend any sort of staging procedures to see if the cancer is still well within the prostate because it invariably will be. On the other hand, if the PSA level is over 10 (some urologists use a cutoff of a PSA level of 20), many urologists will recommend a bone scan to determine if any cancer has spread to bone.

Some urologists like to get abdominal CT scans or magnetic resonance imaging studies with an endorectal coil in place to see if there is any suggestion that the cancer has spread outside the prostate gland (although not necessarily to bone), but most urologists feel that this is an unnecessary study since generally it is not going to affect treatment one way or another. There is no study that will determine with any degree of accuracy whether the pelvic lymph nodes are involved, and this would be the only finding that might impact on the choice of treatment for the prostate cancer. Whether there is an extension of the cancer simply through the prostate capsule would probably not make any difference in the contemplated treatment of prostate cancer, and so, as a general rule, most urologists do not obtain either CT scans or MRI scans as part of their staging workup once the cancer has been diagnosed.

Another factor of considerable importance in planning what to do next is the Gleason sum found on the prostate biopsy. If there is a Gleason sum of 8, 9, or 10, this represents a significantly worse disease than if the Gleason sum is lower. Although I personally feel that a radical prostatectomy may be indicated even in the face of this high Gleason score, many urologists are not at all sanguine about the outcome of any treatment in the face of a high Gleason score. This is something that you and your urologist would have to discuss.

If the option of radiation therapy, either external beam or with the implantation of radioactive seeds into the prostate (or a combination of both), is to be recommended, a patient is usually referred to a radiation therapist who is a specialist in this branch of medicine. As noted in the previous chapter, radiation therapy—external beam, implanted radioactive seeds, or a combination of the two—represents a thoroughly accepted and acceptable alternative to the surgical treatment of prostate cancer. While I personally do not believe that radiation methods of treatment are as effective over the long run as a radical prostatectomy, I always refer every single prostate cancer patient to our radiation therapist so the patient can have a full understanding of that form of therapy and come to an educated decision as to how he wishes to be treated.

Assuming that you, the patient, decide to have a radical prostatectomy, you will be hospitalized the day of surgery and may well have been told to take a bowel preparation medicine at home the night before so the intestines are relatively clean in the very unlikely event of any unplanned damage to the large intestine during the course of the prostatectomy. This is not generally of any serious consequence and it can easily be repaired, but it can be a problem if the bowel has not been properly cleansed prior to the intestinal injury.

The radical prostatectomy itself is a formidable operation (see Chapter 6) that will probably take around two hours, or perhaps longer, including the removal of the pelvic lymph nodes and the prostate. It is usually done under a combination of a spinal and a general anesthetic so you will have complete lower abdominal relaxation and be asleep as well. Following surgery, there is generally only one bladder catheter and it goes through the penis. There is generally a drain left in the lower part of the abdomen that comes out through the skin so that any amount of delayed bleeding and urine leakage can also come out and not collect down in the pelvis. This drain remains inside you for several days or until there is no more drainage. Removal of the drain is not painful. You will be in pain postoperatively, but this pain can usually be controlled by the Patient Controlled Analgesia which was described earlier. Also, at some institutions, an epidural catheter is left in the spinal area to control postoperative discomfort for the first couple of days postoperatively. By the day after surgery (or when the epidural catheter is removed) you will probably be able to sit up in a chair and will, hopefully, be able to take a brief walk, the duration of which will increase each day. Without any doubt, you will have a certain amount of pain and discomfort from this surgery that will require narcotics for its relief. Because of the Patient Controlled Analgesia machines, your postoperative pain and discomfort will be enormously minimized.

The Foley catheter that was placed into your bladder at the time of surgery serves both to drain the bladder during the time of healing and as a splint around which the area where the bladder neck was stitched to the stump of the urethra can heal. I generally like to leave this catheter in place for around two to three weeks following surgery. The presence of the catheter serves to minimize any urine leakage from the area of the repair which might occur since it is extremely difficult to do a watertight repair. It is my practice to send patients home from the hospital following radical prostatectomy two to four days after surgery and to see the patient as an outpatient a couple of weeks later in order to remove the catheter.

When the catheter is removed, most patients will have little or no control whatever over urinary continence and will leak urine to a greater or lesser degree for at least a few days. For this reason a patient is usually given a number of pads that can go inside his shorts to protect his clothing. Within a short period of time, the vast majority of patients recover their continence to the degree that there is not a constant leak while walking around. However, a certain degree of incontinence may remain for several weeks or even months while the entire continence mechanism improves gradually. It may be said that the great majority of patients have little trouble with urine leakage within the time frame of three weeks to three months following surgery. The degree of continence will continue to improve for up to six months or a year after surgery, but if leakage of urine still persists beyond a year, it will probably require definitive therapy (see Chapter 8).

I generally send my patients home with instructions on a specific exercise to restore continence as quickly as possible. This exercise consists of the sequential contraction of two specific muscles. The first is the muscle that the patient used preoperatively when he wanted to suddenly shut off his urinary stream; the second is the muscle that the patient used preoperatively when he wanted to get out that last "squirt" of urine at the time that he thought his voiding was complete. Though these muscles may seem to be the same at first glance, they are actually quite different. I tell my patients to contract the "stop" muscle and immediately contract the so-called squirt muscle and to hold both of these as tightly as possible in a contracted form until unable to hold them any longer because of muscle fatigue. This will usually not be more than ten or fifteen seconds, and I tell the patient to repeat this eight or ten times in a row and to do this eight to ten times each day. In my experience this helps the patient to recover his continence.

The period of convalescence following radical prostatectomy certainly takes longer than the period following surgery for BPH. This is simply because the procedure itself takes much longer and is much more traumatizing to the patient. Within three months you should be feeling as well as you were prior to surgery and able to do all the things you could do prior to surgery. Obviously, with some individuals the time for a full recuperation can be even longer, but this is determined more by the individual than by any variations in the operative procedure.

Many patients want to know about the resumption of sexual activities following radical prostatectomy and particularly whether they are going to be able to achieve erections. As a general rule, it is probably fair and safe to say that if erections are going to return following radical prostate surgery, they will return within six months or a year or, at most, eighteen months postoperatively. Prior to this time one just cannot say whether potency will return. In any case, the operative site is well healed within six weeks following surgery; so sexual activity could safely be resumed at any point after that time if erections are present. Patients must be made aware that they are able to have an orgasm even in the absence of an erection but that they will never again have any ejaculation even with an erection because both the prostate and seminal vesicles have been removed.

When radical prostatectomy is carried out, it is possible sometimes to avoid damaging the nerves on either side of the prostate gland that control erection. Depending on the location of the prostate cancer and its size, it may well be possible to spare one or both of these nerves which control erection. If they are both spared, a patient may well maintain at least partial potency following a radical prostatectomy. If one of them is spared, a patient may still maintain some potency. If neither nerve is spared, a patient may still have some degree of potency although this is unlikely. Another major determination of potency postoperatively, in addition to whether the nerves have been spared, is the patient's age at the time of surgery. Patients over 65 have a considerably lower likelihood of achieving good postoperative erections than younger patients. For those patients who are not able to achieve erections following surgery, the newer forms of penile prosthesis, penile injections, a vacuum pump, or sometimes Viagra represent viable options for erection and ones which are chosen by many patients (see Chapter 8).

Although not generally of any concern to a man having a radical prostatectomy for cancer of the prostate, I should probably note that these patients are permanently infertile following this operation. This is because removal of the entire prostate gland, including the prostatic urethra and the seminal vesicles, precludes having any place for the seminiferous fluid to be made or stored. Recall also that the spermatozoa which enter the prostatic urethra through the ejaculatory ducts via the vas deferens cannot do so because as part of the surgical procedure the vas deferens are tied off. In other words, although a man may have erections and orgasms following a radical prostatectomy, there will be no fluid coming out of the penis.

8

Complications of Prostate Surgery

Surgery for Benign Prostatic Hyperplasia (BPH)

Minimally Invasive Procedures

When treatment with one of the minimally invasive forms of therapy is used, complications are relatively minor. With either the TransUrethral Needle Ablation (TUNA) form of treatment or the microwave thermotherapy (heat treatment) there can be enough edema in the prostate gland immediately following the procedure that voiding is difficult or even impossible. Therefore, with either of these procedures, an indwelling Foley catheter may be necessary in some patients for anywhere from a few hours to a few days. Also, with either of these forms of therapy there may be some discomfort on voiding, but this is usually very minimal and relatively infrequent because the normal urethra is hopefully preserved with both of these forms of minimally invasive therapy. There is a possibility of retrograde ejaculation, but it is not a very common occurrence following either of these minimally invasive procedures. The main "complication" of either of these procedures is that there is no tissue that is removed for the pathologist to examine and so any prostate cancer, if it exists, remains undiscovered. This is not necessarily a problem in older patients (over age 70), but it can be in younger patients in whom definitive treatment for prostate cancer might be indicated if such cancer were discovered.

Vaporization Procedure

With vaporization of the prostate, bleeding can and often does occur during the procedure and this will usually necessitate an indwelling Foley catheter postoperatively for anywhere from overnight to two or three days. The catheter is kept in until the urine is clear of active bleeding. Since the urethral mucosa is effectively destroyed with such a vaporization procedure, many patients will have urgency, frequency, and sometimes discomfort or pain on voiding. These symptoms can last anywhere from a few days to several weeks. Retrograde ejaculation may also be present in some patients.

Laser Treatments

Laser treatment of the prostate gland is now pretty well limited to the interstitial laser which preserves the urethral mucosa and therefore leads to relatively infrequent difficulties with symptoms such as urgency, frequency, or discomfort on voiding, and if any of these symptoms do occur, they are usually short lived. An indwelling catheter is frequently needed for anywhere from overnight to a few days postoperatively in many patients who will have enough edema (swelling) of the prostate gland that voiding becomes very difficult. Also, some patients may have bleeding after an interstitial laser procedure is carried out.

As newer laser procedures come on-line, they will probably have similar postoperative complications to those found with the interstitial laser. The early laser treatments of the prostate involved the so-called side-firing or straight-ahead lasering of the prostate, which destroyed the urethral mucosa and produced up to three months of pronounced voiding discomfort in many patients. For this reason these earlier types of laser treatment of the prostate have pretty much been abandoned. Retrograde ejaculation can also be a complication of a laser treatment of the prostate gland.

TransUrethral Incision of the Prostate (TUIP)

This procedure can also lead to retrograde ejaculation as well as postoperative bleeding. Therefore a catheter is usually required for at least an overnight period and a patient may have some urgency, frequency, and voiding discomfort for a short period of time following surgery. Another "complication" of this procedure, as with the vaporization and the laser procedures, is that no tissue is available for a pathologist to examine, and so any existing prostate cancer will remain undetected.

TransUrethral Resection of the Prostate (TURP)

This procedure remains the gold standard for the surgical treatment of bladder outlet obstruction caused by the prostate gland. It is much harder and more technically difficult to perform than any of the preceding procedures that have been noted for the treatment of BPH, but it also is the one that probably gives the best results for the longest period of time. Even though procedures such as vaporization and lasering of the prostate do appear to give comparable results in the short term, there is just not a long enough follow-up period for these procedures thus far to be able to say how durable any salutary results that are achieved will be.

Postoperative bleeding is certainly a common complication of the TURP, and it is usually treated quite adequately by leaving an indwelling Foley catheter in place until the urine is clear. This is usually anywhere from a few hours to a day or two. Delayed bleeding can also occur, usually brought on by a difficult bowel movement, and this can occur anytime up to three or four weeks postoperatively. It is treated by temporary placement of a Foley catheter.

Incontinence is probably the most-feared and the most-distressing complication of a TURP for both the patient and the physician. The patient is extremely unhappy for the obvious reason that he cannot control his urine, and the physician is equally unhappy because the patient is a walking testimonial to what might appear to be the physician's incompetence. The complication of urinary incontinence is happily an infrequent one but probably does occur in about 1 percent of patients undergoing a TURP for BPH. There are two mechanisms that control urinary continence, and each plays a specific role in maintaining a man in a continent and dry state. One is the musculature that surrounds much of the prostate gland and is outside of the true capsule of the prostate. It serves to maintain the tone of the prostatic urethra and bladder neck and to keep them in a relatively closed position except when the man is voiding. Severe damage to this musculature can lead to profound and total incontinence. The other mechanism for continence is the external urethral sphincter. Damage to this muscle can lead to a stress type of incontinence, which means that there may be an involuntary loss of urine when there is an increased pressure within the abdomen that is transmitted to the bladder. Such pressure can occur with sneezing, coughing, physical exertion, and so on.

Damage to either of these continence mechanisms can occur during the course of the surgery although it may not be recognized at the time. There are very definite landmarks to guide the urologist during the surgical procedure, and whenever surgeon-inflicted damage occurs to the musculature surrounding the prostate gland or to the muscle of the external urethral sphincter, incontinence to a greater or lesser degree may occur. Sometimes vision may be obscured during the course of a transurethral operation because of bleeding, and at other times the problem may result from a relative lack of experience on the part of the urologist. The fact remains that incontinence will still occasionally be a complication in the hands of even the best and most-skilled urologists. The extent of the damage to either continence mechanism will determine the severity of the incontinence; it can vary from a complete and total inability to hold *any* urine in the bladder to a relatively mild loss of urine with severe straining or heavy physical exercise.

When incontinence does occur, of whatever degree, it is not necessarily irreversible or permanent. There are both medical and surgical means of combating this extremely distressing problem. When the urine leakage is due to damage to the musculature surrounding the prostate gland and the prostatic urethra, the undamaged muscle that remains behind can sometimes be stimulated to contract by various drugs and can be brought fairly close to functioning as it did before the surgery. The success or failure of this type of therapy will depend on the extent of damage to the muscles involved and how well the remaining muscles can be made to function. Drugs such as Sudafed or Ephedrine, for example, act on the remaining musculature that surrounds the prostate gland to make it contract, thereby decreasing the inside measurement of the prostatic urethra and promoting continence. Sometimes this medical regime is combined with drug therapy that acts on the bladder to relax it and to minimize its ability to contract (drugs such as Ditropan). This can further help the storage of urine in the bladder and discourage urine leakage to the outside. When the drug therapy is not successful, surgical remedies may well be, but I feel these should not be considered for a minimum of six months and preferably a year after surgery so as to be quite certain that continence will not return spontaneously. The use of a bladder neck "bulking" technique in which collagen is injected into the bladder neck via the transurethral route has also been used to try to treat incontinence, and it has had varying results.

Artificial urinary sphincters, which are usually placed around the urethra just beyond the external urethral sphincter (Fig. 8–1), are also employed and have a very high rate of success. These sphincters look and function like miniature blood pressure cuffs that surround the urethra and totally occlude it when inflated. The sphincters are kept in the inflated state to prevent urinary leakage. When the patient feels that his bladder is filling, he presses the button which is concealed in a pump mechanism buried in the upper part of the scrotum. This deflates that cuff and allows urine to flow freely. Following bladder emptying, the cuff automatically reinflates in about two minutes. These sphincters are certainly not a panacea for all patients, but they are a gigantic step forward in solving this extremely unfortunate problem of postoperative incontinence. Probably somewhere between 75 and 90 percent of patients in whom these prosthetic devices are implanted are able to achieve a very satisfactory degree of continence. Note that these are the same sphincters that are implanted in patients who are incontinent following a radical prostatectomy, and in such cases the sphincter cuff itself is placed around the urethra immediately outside the bladder neck.

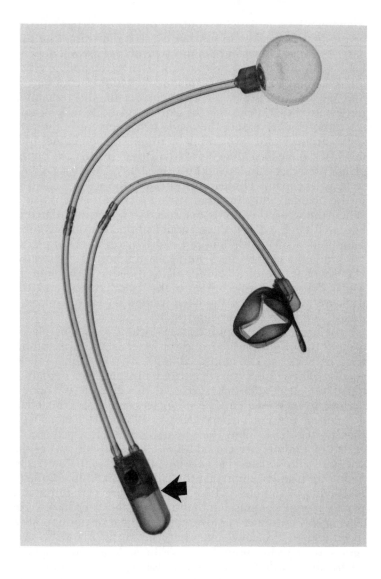

Post-TURP Scarring (Stricture) of the Urethra

This is another complication of transurethral surgery and it is one that is almost totally avoidable. A stricture of the urethra is a scar that can be anywhere in the urethra between the bladder neck and the opening at the end of the penis. However, it is most often found in that part of the urethra where the underside of the penis joins the scrotal skin. It is also commonly found just inside the opening on the end of the penis. This stricture, or narrowing, within the urethra decreases the size of the channel through which the urine flows; so a patient with a significant post-TURP stricture will often have an obstruction to the flow of urine that is as bad or worse than the problem he had that led to the prostate surgery in the first place.

A post-TURP stricture results from trauma to the urethra that may result during the course of the TURP when a patient's urethra is too small for the size of the surgical instrument (the resectoscope) introduced into it. A rough estimate of the frequency of post-TURP strictures can be as high as 10 to 15 percent, although not all of the patients who have these strictures will have any voiding symptoms. They may simply have a urethral channel that is somewhat smaller postoperatively than it was preoperatively. However, the incidence of post-TURP strictures can be reduced to well under 1 percent by measuring the inside of the urethra immediately prior to the insertion of the resectoscope. This is done with a special and very simple instrument. If the inside measurement of the urethra is smaller than a specific size that will vary according

Figure 8–1   *An artificial urinary sphincter. The circular cuff in the center is placed around the urethra just adjacent to the external urethral sphincter. The large, clear reservoir (top) is placed underneath the muscles of the lower abdomen, and the pump mechanism (arrow) is placed in the scrotum. The cuff is kept in the inflated position; when a patient has to urinate, he squeezes a button on the pump that allows fluids to go from the cuff back into the reservoir, thereby deflating the cuff and allowing urine to flow out of the bladder. One or two minutes after the cuff is deflated and the patient has finished voiding, the cuff automatically reinflates.*

to the size of the resectoscope being used, the urethra must be enlarged surgically. This is easily done with another simple instrument that cuts the urethra in its narrowed places so it will not be too small for the resectoscope. After the surgical procedure has been completed, the part of the urethra that has been cut gradually heals and returns to its normal preoperative size.

If a patient does suffer voiding difficulties from a post-TURP stricture, they can sometimes be treated adequately with periodic stretching of the urethra. But sometimes the strictured area must be cut surgically and allowed to heal around a large-sized catheter; this ideally will permit the return of the urethra to its preoperative size. Occasionally, a more extensive plastic surgery operation on the urethra must be done to repair the strictured area.

When one of the open types of surgical operation for BPH has been done (see Chapter 6), a postoperative stricture may result at the spot where the urethra was divided. This is a particular risk if the division of the urethra, which is done as virtually the last step before the obstructing BPH tissue is removed, is not done cleanly and sharply.

Bladder Neck Contracture

This is an infrequent (about 1 percent) but extremely troublesome complication that can occur when very small enlargements of the prostate—the kind of BPH that perhaps does not really warrant surgery—are in fact surgically removed. These very small prostatic enlargements are located entirely within the prostatic urethra and do not extend upward toward the bladder, so they do not cover and protect the normal bladder neck. When operating on these very small prostatic enlargements, therefore, the urologist may find himself cutting away part of the normal bladder neck instead of BPH tissue. The injured bladder neck then tends to heal by scar formation. This will often leave a patient with an extraordinarily small opening in the bladder neck through which the urine must flow. This opening can be as small as a pinhead and will cause the patient to have a recurrence of the symptoms for which he had his prostatic surgery in the first place. The new symptoms, however, are often more severe and pronounced than were those of the prostatic enlargement (BPH). The problem is treated by incising the bladder neck, and this is done through a cystoscope usually with the patient asleep. This cutting may need to be done again because the narrowing of the bladder neck tends to recur. Happily, a bladder neck narrowing is a very infrequent complication of prostatic surgery and is much more easily prevented than treated.

Sexual Problems

These can occur with any of the procedures mentioned for the treatment of BPH but are perhaps more common when a TURP is done than when any of the other procedures are done. Obviously, the ability to achieve an erection that is satisfactory for sexual intercourse is very important to most men. So important, in fact, that many men often delay seeking treatment for medical problems because they fear that the treatment itself may cause them to become impotent. This is often the case with BPH because the myth persists that a man's sex life is over when he has prostate surgery for the relief of BPH. Men, therefore, often delay such surgery to the great detriment of their health and well-being. Moreover, they often enter into the surgery convinced that their sexually active days are behind them. In fact, nothing could be further from the truth, but it is this preconceived notion that may be one of the factors making it so very difficult to accurately assess the true incidence of postoperative loss of erectile function. If such a loss occurs, it may be due to damage from the surgery itself, but it may also be psychogenic because the patient *anticipated* that it would happen.

Another major factor obscuring the cause and effect relationship of surgery for BPH and postoperative impotence is the fact that *any* surgery can have a deleterious effect on erectile function, an effect probably due to a combination of psychogenic and organic stimuli from the general bodily insult that results from any surgical procedure and not to specific damage to the structures that affect potency. Having said all of the foregoing, however, the fact remains that between 10 and 20 percent of men having a TURP will indeed claim that they were potent preoperatively and unable to achieve an erection postoperatively. The figures for erectile dysfunction following any of the surgical procedures for BPH other than a TURP are not well known, but there may well be an incidence of impotence following these less invasive procedures. The nerves affecting impotence do closely invest the prostate gland on either side, and it is conceivable that one or both of these nerves may be damaged if a resection is carried too deeply or if heat transferred through the prostate when a vaporization or a laser procedure is used damages these nerves. In any case, if the patient does indeed have postoperative erectile dysfunction, it is treated in much the same manner as erectile dysfunction that occurs unrelated to prostate surgery.

There are several methods that are widely used for the treatment of erectile dysfunction that occurs after prostatic surgery that is done either for benign prostatic hyperplasia or for prostate cancer (a radical prostatectomy). Furthermore, these same modalities are usedN for erectile dysfunction that occurs unrelated to any prostate surgery. Perhaps the most popular method now in use involves the oral medication that goes by the trade name of Viagra. This is a pill that acts through an enzymatic system to increase the effects of nitric oxide, a substance that is crucial to the erectile mechanism within the penis, and it is effective in about 75 percent of men who use it. The pill is taken about an hour before intercourse is desired, and one-half hour following this, manual or oral stimulation of the penis must be carried out. A patient cannot simply take the pill, sit back, and get an erection. The erection should then last for about a half hour and the most common side effects are headache and visual disturbances such that the patient thinks he is looking through a pair of blue-green sunglasses.

This drug is absolutely contraindicated in any patient who is taking any form of nitrates such as nitroglycerin. I believe it is also extremely unwise to use in any patient with any cardiac disease although I have not infrequently referred my patients to a cardiologist for a clearance to take Viagra if they were not on any nitroglycerin or other nitrates but simply had some history of heart trouble. Quite simply, Viagra tends to lower blood pressure and this is exactly what nitroglycerin and other nitrates do. If by any chance Viagra is taken concomitantly with a nitrate, the blood pressure can drop sharply enough to induce a heart attack, and it is a fact that several hundred people have already been reported to have died as a result of taking this Viagra medication.

Another very popular form of therapy for erectile dysfunction is the injection of prostaglandin E1 directly into the corpus cavernosum of the penis. This will induce an erection, following manual stimulation of the penis, in about 80 percent or more of men. The erection can last for an hour or so and it is a very satisfactory form of treatment for many men. The biggest risk involved is that the patient may inject too much of the medication and can then wind up with a condition known as priapism which is a prolonged, painful, and inappropriate erection that needs to be treated by injecting an antidote directly into the penis, something that usually requires an emergency room visit.

Another form of treatment for erectile dysfunction is the use of a vacuum device (Fig. 8–2). This is a cylinder into which the flaccid penis is placed. The air is then manually pumped out of the cylinder. This results in an erection which may be maintained for up to a half-hour by means of a constricting band which is placed around the base of the penis just before the penis is removed from the cylinder. The cost of these vacuum devices is in the neighborhood of $150 to $400. Still another type of treatment for erectile dysfunction is the use of a small pellet that is inserted into the urethra by means of a special applicator. The applicator system is known as MUSE which stands for Medicated Urethral System for Erection, and the pellet introduced into the urethra contains prostaglandin E1. After the pellet is inserted, the penis is massaged to promote absorption of the pellet. This system seems to bring satisfactory results to about 30 to 50 percent of men who try it, but about 10 percent of men who try it complain of a burning sensation in the penis.

Alternative and more permanent forms of therapy involve the implantation of one of the various kinds of penile prostheses. These are devices that go into the spongy bodies of the penis (the corpora cavernosa) and stiffen them to allow penetration during intercourse. Although there are many different brands of penile prostheses, the two fundamental types are the semirigid and the inflatable (Figures 8–3 and 8–4). Each of these has several advantages, and the ultimate decision as to which type to use is properly a decision made jointly by the patient and his urologist.

Newer forms of therapy for erectile dysfunction will undoubtedly be coming on-line. Approval by the Federal Drug Administration is anticipated momentarily for an apo-

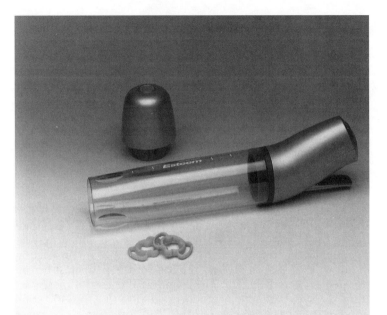

Figure 8–2   *The vacuum pump used to produce an erection. This is known as the Erec-aid and pictured in the middle is the cylinder into which the penis is placed. At the right side of the cylinder is the hand-operated pump, which creates a vacuum within the cylinder and produces an erection. At the bottom of the picture are the compression bands that are loaded onto the cylinder and then placed around the base of the penis to maintain the erection. At the top of the photograph, the small cylindrical device is a loader used for the purpose of conveniently placing the compression bands onto the cylinder. (Photograph courtesy of Timm Medical Technologies, Inc., Eden Prairie, Minnesota.)*

morphine product that will be marketed as Uprima. This is a sublingual (under the tongue) tablet that works in about five minutes to produce an erection. It works on the erection center in the brain, but in its clinical trials it has induced nausea in some people and syncope in others. It probably is not any better than Viagra except for the fact that it should work much more rapidly and hopefully there will be no nitrate contraindications such as exist with Viagra. However, some

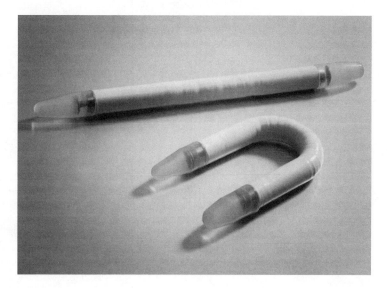

Figure 8–3 *A semirigid (malleable) penile prosthesis. This type of prosthesis has virtually no working parts that can break or malfunction. Although the penis is always rigid, the patient is able to bend his penis so that it points downward along the inner part of his thigh and does not interfere with usual daily activity. When intercourse is desired, the penis can be bent upward so that it sticks straight out. To illustrate this, the photograph shows only one of what would normally be the two paired prostheses in the rigid position and also as it is bent in the downward position. This is to illustrate its flexibility and its ease of concealment. (Photograph courtesy of Timm Medical Technologies, Inc., Eden Prairie, Minnesota.)*

concern has been raised, because of the syncope in some patients, that the concomitant use of nitrates could have a deleterious effect on the heart should syncope occur. Syncope can be considered to be almost like fainting but usually without the loss of consciousness.

Some companies are working on drugs that are similar to Viagra in their action but without any nitrate contraindications, and still other companies are working on topical prostaglandin (PGE1) which would be applied to the glans penis. It would be combined with skin enhancers to promote absorption but yet would not have any long-term effects. There are

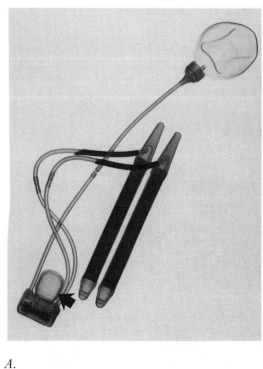

A.

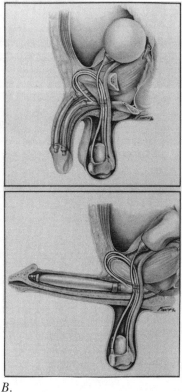

B.

Figure 8–4 INFLATABLE PROSTHESIS
This type of prosthesis allows for an increase of girth, as well as rigidi-
ty of the penis when the device is inflated; it also allows for a normal
flaccid state of the penis when the device is deflated. (Illustrations
courtesy of American Medical Systems, Minnetonka, Minnesota.)
  A. The most-frequently used inflatable device, in which the
pump (arrow) that is placed within the scrotum is squeezed, thereby
transferring fluid from the reservoir (top of photograph) into the
paired cylinders, making the penis increase in girth and rigidity.*
When the erection is no longer desired, a release valve on the pump
permits the transfer of fluid from the cylinders back into the reservoir.
  B. An artist's drawing showing where the various parts of the
inflatable device illustrated in Panel A are placed anatomically. Top:
the penis is flaccid and the prosthesis deflated. Bottom: the penis is
erect and the prosthesis is inflated. Note the increase in the size of the
cylinders when the penis is rigid, and the corresponding decrease in
the size of the reservoir since much of the fluid has been transferred
from the reservoir to the cylinders.
  *Note that there are other models of the inflatable prosthesis that
vary slightly from that which is shown, but the principle is the same.

at least two companies working on this and the product may be available in the near future.

Another new treatment that should be approved by the time this book is published is a penile injection that will use a combination of phentolamine and vasoactive intestinal polypeptide. The advantage of this in clinical trials has been that it causes less penile discomfort than does the Caverjet injections (prostaglandin E1).

Perhaps most exciting is research that is going on in the field of gene therapy to enable the penis to make more nitric oxide. It is postulated that perhaps an injection once a year might significantly enhance a patient's ability to achieve erections. This, however, is not likely to be available in the immediate or even near future.

Retrograde Ejaculation

Retrograde ejaculation is the term used when a man has an orgasm and climaxes but nothing comes out of the urethra. Normally, at the time of ejaculation, the bladder neck closes, and the semen is propelled to the outside by the spasmodic contractions of the muscles surrounding the urethra. However, after transurethral surgery that is done to relieve prostatic obstruction, the bladder neck is enlarged to the point that it may not close at the time of climax and ejaculation, and so the semen takes the path of least resistance and goes backward into the bladder. It may then be noted within the urine when a patient voids following his orgasm. When a patient has had a TransUrethral Resection of the Prostate (TURP), this retrograde ejaculation is a very common occurrence and probably a majority of patients that have a TURP wind up with retrograde ejaculation after surgery. With some of the other surgical treatments for benign prostatic hyperplasia, the bladder neck may not be enlarged to the degree that it is opened during a TURP and therefore the incidence of retrograde ejaculation is lower than it would be following a TURP. Indeed, retrograde ejaculation would be far less common with, for example, microwave thermotherapy or a TransUrethral Incision of the Prostate (TUIP) than it is with some of the other procedures that are more likely to enlarge the opening at the bladder neck.

For most patients retrograde ejaculation does not diminish the pleasurable sensation of an orgasm, and the feeling that accompanies an orgasm is, for most people, unchanged. However, it is absolutely imperative that a patient be advised of the distinct possibility, perhaps even the probability, of retrograde ejaculation occurring following surgery for BPH. I can well remember the very first TURP I did after finishing my residency program. My patient was a gentleman in his late seventies. I failed to make any comment to him prior to surgery about retrograde ejaculation, and when it happened to him following his surgery, he was extremely angry! "You have taken away my manhood!" he told me with considerable distress. The fact that the gentleman was not married and had no desire to have any children had nothing to do with it. I think this gets to the crux of what is so distressing to men about retrograde ejaculation. It is simply the idea that *if* they wanted to have children this would no longer be possible. Somehow or other the idea that pervades the brain of some men is that removing the possibility of fatherhood makes them less of a man. This is something I find difficult to comprehend, but it remains a fact. I can well remember the anguish of a good friend of mine, an attorney, who had never married and had always abhorred the presence of little children but who was nevertheless extremely irate with his retrograde ejaculation that followed a TURP. He truly felt that the absence of an ejaculate robbed him of one of the paramount hallmarks of being a man, and there was little I could do to convince him otherwise. Happily, he was not my patient and so the brunt of his anger was not directed at me!

In the event a retrograde ejaculation does occur in an individual who is intent on fathering more children, there are techniques that are readily available to isolate the semen from the urine which is voided immediately after ejaculation. These techniques are neither difficult nor exotic, and the semen that is recovered can be injected into the vagina, in close proximity to the cervix, in the same manner that artificial insemination is done.

I indicated above that the great majority of patients who have retrograde ejaculation following surgery still have the same pleasurable sensation that they had prior to surgery. However, I have learned from some very few of my patients that this is not uniformly the case. Very uncommonly, patients will complain that the feeling during orgasm following surgery for BPH was "just different" and the different feeling "not nearly as good as it was before." Even though I know from experience with many patients over many years that such a reaction represents the findings of a very small number of patients, I do feel it important to relate this potential problem to you. One very upset patient's wife wrote a letter to me to say that her husband, since his TURP, took an extraordinarily long time to reach a climax and was not able to do so on every occasion. I am unable to account for such situations as these, but I certainly do not doubt the accurate description of these situations as told to me by these very troubled patients. I do, however, want to reiterate to you that although these problems can and do occur, the great majority of patients who have prostate surgery for BPH do indeed return to the same sexual patterns, practices, sensation, and feeling that they had prior to the surgery (except for the retrograde ejaculation).

Epididymitis

This is a complication of prostate surgery that may occur while a patient is in the hospital, but it usually occurs two to six weeks following surgery when the patient is well on his way to recovery at home. It is a condition in which there is a pronounced inflammation and enlargement of the epididymis (Chapter 1) accompanied by considerable pain and tenderness. The inflammatory process not infrequently also involves the adjacent testis producing a large, hard, extremely tender mass within the scrotum that can be as large as a plum or even a small peach. Epididymitis is a most uncommon complication of prostate surgery that probably occurs in 1 to 2 percent of patients, and it is most likely to occur if a patient had infected urine preoperatively or a prior history of epididymitis. When it does occur, the acute discomfort usually goes away in one to two weeks but the swelling can take up to two or three months to resolve completely. Treatment is with antibiotics, pain medications, and rest. A scrotal support is also helpful.

Persistent Bacteriuria

Following prostatic surgery for benign disease it takes two to three months before the prostatic urethra has formed its new lining assuming that the procedure was one in which the normal urethra was destroyed. This would be the case with a vaporization of the prostate, with a TURP, and with some of the laser procedures. The lining of the bladder subsequently grows downward into the prostatic urethra to form a new lining. During this period when the area of the prostatic urethra is healing, there is a constant shedding of white blood cells (pus cells). This is a normal part of the healing process. It does not mean that infection is necessarily present. So, even though there are many white blood cells in the urine of patients recovering from prostate surgery, it does not necessarily mean that any bacterial infection is present in the urine. Indeed, if bacteria *are* present in the urine of patients who are recovering from prostatic surgery, it is abnormal and should be treated.

The usual treatment consists of several days of an antibiotic to which the bacteria are susceptible. If it is not possible to sterilize the urine by this means or if the infection recurs after successful treatment, then a thorough investigation is necessary to look for those causes of infection which may have been overlooked and which generally require further treatment. Such things as incomplete bladder emptying, which may or may not be due to incomplete removal of obstructing BPH tissue, bladder diverticulae (outpouchings usually caused by BPH, see Chapter 4) that do not empty, and even obstruction to the drainage of a kidney that has bacteria in it can all result in recurrent infection following prostatic surgery. Occasionally, kidney stones that were not known about prior to the surgery can be the source of the bacterial infection. When the reason for the infection is found, treatment can usually correct it. Some urologists prefer to keep patients on antibiotics for several weeks following surgery whereas others prefer to treat infections if they occur. While I tend to agree with the latter, it may certainly be said that there is no right or wrong in this issue, and a physician will generally follow the course that he or she has found to be the most successful in the past.

Surgery for Cancer of the Prostate

Transurethral Surgery

Complications that can occur when a transurethral prostatic operation is done for a patient with prostatic cancer who has symptoms of bladder outlet obstruction due to a coexisting BPH are the same as those that can occur when the operation is done for BPH alone. This is particularly true when the obstructing tissue is predominantly benign. This is a common occurrence, since, you will recall, cancer of the prostate and BPH both occur in the same age group.

However, if the transurethral surgery is done to relieve the obstructive symptoms caused by an advanced cancer of the prostate, then the complications of the surgery are much more severe. This is because when the entire prostate (or most of it) has been replaced by cancerous tissue, the prostatic urethra becomes more of a rigid tube and not at all pliable. Since one of the mechanisms for continence depends on the pliability of the prostatic urethra, so that it can virtually close off this channel at times, it is obvious that if the cancer turns the prostatic urethra into a rigid structure, continence could become a real problem. Incontinence of urine does, in fact, occur in 5 percent or even more of patients who have a TURP to relieve the obstructive symptoms of advanced prostatic cancer. The likelihood of incontinence increases if the patient has additionally had radiation therapy for the treatment of his prostate cancer. Bleeding following TURP for advanced cancer of the prostate can also be a formidable problem because there are certain substances in the cancerous tissue itself that tend to promote bleeding and prevent the usual process of blood coagulation through which bleeding usually stops. Finally, it should be recalled that a TURP of the prostate with advanced and extensive malignancy (or even a TURP done for BPH and coexisting cancer) must be looked on as a purely palliative procedure to alleviate voiding difficulties, and it certainly is never to be considered as a cure for the cancer.

Radical (Total) Prostatectomy

Incontinence When a radical prostatectomy is done in an attempt to achieve a cure or a long-term survival in a patient with prostate cancer, the entire prostate gland is removed along with the prostatic urethra (see Chapter 6). A gap in the continuity of the urethra is obviously created. This is bridged by bringing the bladder neck down to the remaining portion of the urethra at the level of the external urethral sphincter. The bladder neck is then stitched to that remaining stump of the urethra. Obviously, therefore, when the entire prostate and its musculature is removed, there is always going to be a chance of urinary incontinence even if the reconstruction of the urethra is perfectly done. In fact, between 5 and 10 percent of patients undergoing radical prostatectomy nationwide do suffer from a pronounced degree of incontinence. However, certain centers that perform very large numbers of radical prostatectomies report continence rates that approach 100 percent. Virtually all patients who have had a radical prostatectomy are totally incontinent for anywhere from a few hours to a few days or even a few weeks or possibly a few months following radical prostatectomy, but only in a very few patients (something over 5 percent) is this incontinence permanent. About one-third of patients who have a radical prostatectomy can have some degree of stress incontinence for a prolonged period of time or even permanently. This means that when these patients cough or sneeze or lift something, they may involuntarily lose anywhere from a few drops to several centimeters of urine. Most of these patients need to wear protective pads. This situation can be helped by drugs which relax the bladder and make it less susceptible to voiding urges. Such drugs as Ditropan, Detrol, and Imipramine are frequently helpful.

Since one of the principal mechanisms for continence (the entire prostate gland with its accompanying muscles) has been removed during a radical prostatectomy, the regaining of continence is dependent in large part on the diligent use of an exercise. This means the patient himself must embark on a regular schedule of doing the exercise to add tone and strength to the remaining muscles that control continence. There are actually two groups of muscles that are used, the first of which is around the rectum and the second which is around the base of the penis. The first is the muscle group that you tightened when you suddenly wanted to stop the flow of urine while you were voiding; think back to when you used to urinate prior to your radical prostatectomy. The second of these muscle groups is the one you would use when you thought you were all through voiding and you wanted to expel the last few drops, or the last squirt, of urine.

The exercise to improve continence is to contract these two groups of muscles sequentially starting with the one you would use to stop the flow of urine while voiding and then, while keeping that group of muscles contracted, additionally contracting the group of muscles that you would use to get out the last squirt of urine at the end of voiding. You should hold both of these groups of muscles in a contracted state—as tightly as you can—for as long as you possibly can until they fatigue. In practice, this will not be more than ten or fifteen seconds. You should repeat this exercise—contracting both groups of muscles sequentially—at least eight or ten times in a row and you should do this eight or ten times a day. You should also make a conscious effort to contract these muscles, again sequentially, before lifting, straining, or doing anything that might place an increased pressure on your bladder and result in an involuntary loss of urine.

In the course of the healing process after a radical prostatectomy, improvement in regaining continence can be anticipated for up to a year or even eighteen months following surgery. If the incontinence of urine is still sufficient to cause distress to a patient beyond that point, there are various treatments that can be implemented. The injection of a bulking substance such as collagen directly into the bladder neck (done transurethrally) often greatly improves continence, but its effects are not always long lasting and the collagen injections frequently need to be repeated. An artificial sphincter can be surgically implanted as already described for the incontinence that can result from surgery for BPH. These artificial sphincters, when used following a radical prostatectomy, are placed around the bladder neck. While certainly not totally effective in all patients, these artificial sphincters do indeed provide significant improvement and sometimes total cure in a majority of patients in whom they are implanted.

Contracture of the Bladder Neck Contracture of the bladder neck in the area where it is stitched to the remaining portion of the urethra is a not infrequent complication of radical prostate surgery. It occurs within the first three months after the operation. Typically, the patient will note that his urinary stream diminishes in force and caliber sharply and he has difficulty voiding. These are the same symptoms as those of a bladder neck contracture following prostatic surgery for BPH. Treatment can sometimes be as simple as a dilation of the bladder neck which is carried out transurethrally under local anesthetic, but sometimes the contracture is so small that it has to be incised under a general or a spinal anesthetic. As a general rule, either the dilation or the incision is sufficient to relieve the problem, and it is uncommon for this particular complication of bladder neck contracture to persist or to recur once it has been treated.

Erectile Dysfunction When the nerves that control erection are spared during the radical prostatectomy, erectile function may remain adequate postoperatively. However, these nerves are in close contact with the prostate gland on either side and there are many urologists who feel it is not always a wise thing to do to try to preserve these nerves for fear that that may, in fact, be preserving some of the cancer that might have been out in the periphery of the prostate gland. It is also a fact that many patients undergoing radical prostatectomy are no longer potent prior to the surgery and so the sparing of these nerves is not important. Nevertheless, when postoperative potency is indeed important to a patient, it can sometimes be preserved by sparing these nerves, and you and your urologist should discuss this point very carefully giving careful credence to the opinion of your urologist as to whether such nerve sparing runs the risk of sparing any cancer that might be close to or even adherent to these nerves.

Sometimes, when prostate biopsies show cancer only on one side of the prostate gland, the sparing of the nerve on the other side is a valid option although sparing only one nerve does not produce the firm erection that sparing both nerves may often produce. Also, the age of the patient at the time of surgery is a major factor in how potent he will be following surgery. In general, patients much over 65 years of age do not tend to remain potent postoperatively even when the nerves are spared. There is no doubt that there are some urologists with a vast experience in doing radical prostatectomies, and these urologists report a potency rate of 75 percent or more in their patients who have had nerve-sparing radical prostatectomies. Some excellent surgical centers report an even higher percentage of retained potency in men under 60 and better than 80 to 85 percent of men overall retaining potency one to two years after surgery. Most centers, however, are not able to report such good results, and nationwide data suggest that about 40 to 50 percent of men of all ages have retained potency one to two years after a nerve-sparing radical prostatectomy. Potency rates, of course, are lower when there has been no nerve sparing.

Impotence following a radical prostatectomy may be temporary or it may be permanent. If potency is going to return, it should do so within a year or eighteen months following surgery. Beyond that point, if impotency persists, it can be treated in the same manner as when it occurs following surgery for BPH. The Viagra pills are sometimes effective following prostatectomy, but their success rate is much lower in this situation than when they are used following surgery for BPH. If there has been nerve sparing on one or both sides, Viagra is more likely to work. However, the vacuum pump and the penile injections are indeed helpful in most cases. The intraurethral MUSE system may also be helpful. Where none of these measures seems to help, implanting a penile prosthesis, as noted previously, will usually solve the problem.

The impotence often associated with prostate cancer, and indeed the prostate cancer itself, are often understandably the cause of great concern and anxiety to many men. For some, the presence of a support group of men who have been through a similar experience may be most helpful. There are several support groups in this country for men with prostate cancer; perhaps the largest and best known is an organization known as "Us Too." This organization has many chapters throughout North America (most of them in the United States) and you can find the telephone number of the one nearest you by calling 1-800-242-2383. This is the telephone number of the American Foundation for Urologic Disease and that organization can help you locate the chapter nearest to you.

Some General Comments

A radical prostatectomy is a formidable operation and a difficult one to perform, and not all urologists are able to achieve the same results. I do believe that a well-trained urologist who performs many of these operations with care and skill will achieve better results in terms of fewer postoperative complications, a lessened likelihood of incontinence, and a greater likelihood of preservation of potency than will another urologist who perhaps is not as well trained and who does not do as many radical prostatectomies. There is nothing new in this statement which I just made. It is a given that excellent surgeons will usually get better results, with fewer complications, than poorer surgeons. One of the factors distinguishing excellent surgeons from poorer surgeons is the high volume of a given surgical procedure that they do. Therefore, I believe that your surgery is likely to have fewer complications and perhaps even a lesser chance of your being incontinent, if you go to a urologist or to an institution that has great experience with this type of surgery. I hasten to add, however, that some of the very excellent urologists with whom I have come in contact over the years do not work in large institutions and do not necessarily have the largest number of surgical cases under their belts.

The kinds of complications discussed in this chapter that can occur when prostate surgery is done either for benign prostatic hyperplasia or for cancer are not common, but they certainly can and do occur. In the present day atmosphere it is generally accepted that informed patients who fully understand their surgery often do better postoperatively and have better results. Moreover, a patient is *entitled* to know and understand a surgical procedure. For these reasons the concept of informed consent is one that has gained wide acceptance in medical and legal circles. This simply means that when a patient gives his consent for an operation, he has been informed about what the operation is, what the risks are, and what the potential complications are. It is sometimes a difficult balancing act for a urologist to determine just exactly how much detail a patient may want to know—or should know— about the risks and complications of surgery. Unquestionably, a presentation covering every conceivably bad thing that might happen to a patient and covering it in lurid detail might well scare the patient away from needed surgery or might send the patient into a surgical procedure with enormous apprehension about possible complications. On the other hand, it is unquestionably a patient's right to know about the things that might go wrong with an operation so he can have the opportunity to refuse the surgery if he wants to.

When I am discussing the subject of risks and complications with my patients, I will always answer in an honest and forthright way any questions that they ask me and I will be as frank with my patients as I would want my own doctor to be with me. However, I do not think it particularly wise or helpful to a patient to scare him before an operation by bringing up things that are most unlikely to happen, particularly when these are things that the patient has never even considered. Most of my patients want to know what the risks are in terms of mortality, and I tell them this truthfully, to the best of my knowledge. Most of my patients also want to know about the possibility of incontinence and I answer this as truthfully as I can. Some of my patients ask about the sexual activity they may anticipate following surgery and I always explain this in great detail; in fact, this is one subject that I will bring up if a patient fails to ask anything about it.

Radiation Therapy

Not infrequently patients will select radiation therapy, external beam, implantation of radioactive seeds, or a combination of the two, as a treatment of choice for prostatic cancer. Sometimes the complications of this form of treatment can be every bit as significant to the patient as the complications of radical surgery.

About half the patients undergoing any form of radiation therapy for prostate cancer may ultimately suffer from erectile dysfunction and impotence as a result of the therapy, and it is *not* psychogenic impotence. The precise mechanism responsible for this loss of erectile function is not well understood, but it is probably related to the effect of the radiation on the blood vessels supplying the spongy parts of the penis. Treatment of this erectile dysfunction has the same options as listed earlier in this chapter. Unfortunately, a very small percent of patients undergoing radiation therapy (about 2 percent) will have severe complications such as uncontrollable bladder hemorrhages (which usually occur some years after the radiation therapy has been completed), urinary incontinence, or significant damage to the rectum. About 5 percent of patients undergoing radiation therapy will have more moderate complications and these usually affect the bladder or the rectum. As I noted in Chapter 6, I always offer my patients the opportunity to visit with our radiation therapist to get a far better understanding about the benefits, risks, and complications of radiation therapy than I am able to offer them. I would encourage you, the patient, to ask your urologist for this same option of discussing your treatment with a radiation therapist unless you already know (as some patients do) that radiation therapy is not the treatment you personally want to have.

Postorchiectomy Complications

Patients undergoing this procedure for the treatment of advanced prostate cancer almost never have any problems with feminization such as breast enlargement, voice change, or changes in bodily or facial hair distribution. However, many patients complain bitterly about "hot flashes," a problem that leaves many men dripping wet with perspiration several times each day. This is quite analogous to the hot flashes that women undergo during menopause. Although a majority of patients having an orchiectomy (or being treated with LH-RH agonist injections) do not have this severe problem with hot flashes, the problem is a very real and significant one for those who do.

I have found that there are three treatments to deal with this problem, any one of which may be successful for a given patient. The intramuscular injection of medroxyprogesterone acetate (Provera) in a dosage of 200 to 400 milligrams every four to six weeks often greatly alleviates the problem. Sometimes oral Premarin (this is a conjugated estrogen) in a dose of 0.3 to 0.6 milligrams a day by mouth helps. Another medication that is very helpful but can be quite costly is Bellergal-S, one capsule twice a day. Most patients can be greatly helped, if not cured, of this distressing problem of hot flashes by one of these forms of therapy. I usually start with the Provera because that is relatively long acting and the patient only needs to repeat the injections every four to six weeks and sometimes not even that often.

A Last Word to My Readers

I do hope that this book has been helpful to you as you struggle with any of the problems concerning your prostate gland. I have tried in this book to cover virtually all of the situations that might arise and that might concern you, and I hope that I have been successful in doing this. I would also like to thank the many readers whose written and telephone communications to me following earlier editions of this book have helped to form some of the basis for the material in this present book.

Finally, I want to repeat what I have said in the Introduction of this book, and that is that different physicians who are equally capable and equally intelligent may well follow different diagnostic routes to the same end and may well use different methods for treating the same disease. None of these physicians is necessarily wrong, for the differences merely reflect the fact that in the hands of a given physician one treatment has consistently shown better results than another and physicians will have differing experiences that will lead to different conclusions. Throughout this book, I frequently have expressed my own opinions about the diagnosis and treatment of many urologic problems. However, my opinions are just that and certainly are not meant to imply in any way that others who may differ with me are wrong.

I do hope that this book has fulfilled the expectations of those who have read it; I will be most satisfied if it has served to comfort and to reassure those men suffering from the various diseases of the prostate gland.

GLOSSARY

Accessory sex gland   a mass of glandular tissue that plays a peripheral (not primary) role in procreation.

Acid phosphatase   an enzyme made in the prostate gland.

Acute   reaching a crisis rapidly; having a short and relatively severe course; sharp; poignant.

Acute bacterial prostatitis   *see* Prostatitis, bacterial, acute.

Adenoma   a benign tumor in which the cells form recognizable glandular structures.

Adenomatous enlargement   pertaining to the growth of adenoma.

Alkaline phosphatase   an enzyme produced in the liver, the bone, and other structures.

American Board of Urology   Organized in 1934, the board's purpose is to serve the public by ascertaining the competency of any physician who is specializing or who wishes to specialize in the field of urology. It arranges and conducts examinations testing the qualifications of voluntary candidates, issues certificates to accepted candidates duly licensed by law (and also holds the power to revoke certificates), and prepares lists of the urologists whom it has certified.

Anesthesia   a loss of feeling or sensation. Although the term is used for loss of tactile sensibility, it is applied especially to loss of the sensation of pain, as it is induced to permit performance of surgery or other painful procedures.

General   a state of unconsciousness, produced by anesthetic agents, with absence of pain sensation over the entire body and a greater or lesser degree of muscle relaxation.

Local   confined to one part of the body.

Spinal   produced by an injection of a local anesthetic into the subarachnoid space around the spinal cord.

Artificial urinary sphincter   a prosthesis designed to restore continence in an incontinent person by constricting the urethra.

Aspiration   the removal of fluids or gases from a cavity by the application of suction.

Needle   removal of cell samples with suction from a specially designed needle which is attached to a syringe.

Prostatic   removal of cell or tissue samples from the prostate gland.

Bacteria   unicellular microorganisms that may be harmful to humans and may cause infection or inflammation.

Bacterial localization tests   tests devised to isolate the focus of a bacterial infection in order to appropriately treat the infection. A common test is to determine if there is bacterial infection in the prostate or the urethra.

Bacterial prostatitis   *see* Prostatitis, bacterial.

Bacteriuria   the presence of bacteria in the urine.

Benign   not malignant; not recurrent; favorable for recovery.

Benign Prostatic Hyperplasia (BPH)   the nonmalignant but abnormal multiplication of the number of normal cells in prostatic tissue.

Benign prostatic hypertrophy (BPH)   overgrowth of the prostate due to an increase in size of its constituent cells, as opposed to hyperplasia which is the multiplication of those cells. *See also* Benign prostatic hyperplasia.

Biopsy   the removal and examination, usually microscopic, of tissue from the living body, which is performed to establish a precise diagnosis.

Bladder   a sac, such as one serving as a receptacle for a secretion. Often used alone to designate the urinary bladder.

Bladder catheterization   passage of a catheter into the urinary bladder.

Bladder neck contracture   an abnormal narrowing of the bladder neck such that the urine passage is hindered. Can be a complication of prostate surgery.

Bladder outlet   the first portion of the natural channel through which urine flows when it leaves the bladder.

Bladder outlet obstruction   obstruction of the bladder outlet causing problems with urination or the retention of urine in the bladder. *See also* Bladder outlet.

Bladder spasm   a sudden and involuntary contraction of the bladder muscle(s), often attended by pain and interference with bladder function.

Bladder trigone   the most dependent and most sensitive part of the bladder. Located at the base of the bladder near the bladder neck.

Blastic lesion   *see* Lesion, blastic.

Blood urea nitrogen (BUN)   a blood test to measure kidney function.

Bone scans   *see* Scans, bone.

Bone x-rays   x-rays of the bones.

Bulbous urethra   *see* Urethra, bulbous.

Cancer   a cellular tumor, the natural course of which is fatal. Cancer cells, unlike benign tumor cells, exhibit the properties of invasion and metastases.

Capsule   the structure in which something is enclosed.

Carcinoma   a malignant new growth made up of epithelial cells tending to infiltrate the surrounding tissues and giving rise to metastases.

Catheter   a tubular, flexible, surgical instrument for withdrawing fluids from (or introducing fluids into) a cavity of the body, especially one for introduction into the bladder through the urethra for the withdrawal or urine.

Chlamydia   a family of small spherical-shaped bacterial organisms that commonly cause infection in the urethra.

Chronic bacterial prostatitis   the persistence over a long period of time of bacterial prostatitis (infection).

Compensated bladder   a bladder that empties completely on voiding.

Computed tomography (CT) scanning   the imaging technique combining x-rays with computer technology to provide a cross-section image.

Continuous, or indwelling, catheterization   catheterization in which the patient has a catheter in place for a protracted length of time.

Contracture, bladder neck   *see* Bladder neck contracture.

Creatinine   a normal metabolic waste product the measurement of which in the blood is used as an excellent parameter of kidney function.

Cystoscope   an instrument used for the examination of the interior of the urinary bladder and urethra.

Cystoscopy   direct visual examination of the urinary tract with a cystoscope.

Cytology   the study of cells: their origin, structure, function, and pathology.

Decompensated bladder   a bladder that does not empty when voiding so that residual urine remains after voiding.

Detrusor   the smooth muscle forming the muscular wall of the urinary bladder. On contraction it serves to expel the urine.

Digital rectal examination (prostate)   examination of the prostate by insertion of the index finger into the rectum.

Diverticulum   a pouch or sac branching out from a hollow organ structure such as the bladder.

Dribbling, terminal   an involuntary loss of urine at the conclusion of voiding that occurs in drops or in an unsteady stream.

Ejaculate   the semen expelled in a single ejaculation.

Ejaculatory duct   the tubular passage through which the semen reaches the prostatic urethra during orgasm.

Enucleation   the removal of an organ, a tumor, or another body in such a way that it comes out clean and whole, like a nut from its shell.

Enzyme-linked immunoassay   a type of laboratory test in which an enzyme level is determined using an immunological assay.

Epididymis   an elongated, cordlike structure along the posterior border of the testis that provides storage, transit, and maturation of sperm.

Epididymitis   inflammation of the epididymis.

Epithelium   the covering of internal and external surfaces of the body, including the lining of blood vessels and other small cavities.

Erectile dysfunction   impaired or disordered function of the penis regarding its role in vaginal penetration. Also called impotence.

Estrogen therapy   the use of estrogen to lower the circulating androgen level to castrate level in the palliative treatment of prostate cancer.

Excretory urogram (IVP)   *see* X-rays.

External urethral sphincter   the ringlike band of muscle fibers that voluntarily constricts the passage of urine from the bladder to the outside.

False negative   the erroneous result of a test that is reported as negative but is truly positive.

False positive   the erroneous result of a test that is reported as positive but is truly negative.

Family physician the doctor who cares for the family as a whole, usually treating the family unit where appropriate and making referrals to specialists as indicated.

First-glass urine the first glass used in a study of the urine in which three glasses are used in all to determine prostate infection as opposed to bladder or urethral infection.

Flow rate (urine) the measurement of urine as it is expelled from the bladder at its peak period of movement. If this measurement is lower than normal values, it shows that obstruction may be present.

Foley catheter a catheter which is placed into the bladder for continuous drainage and which is kept in place by means of a balloon that is inflated with liquid within the bladder.

Fossa a hollowed out place.

Frequency the desire to urinate at close intervals.

Gallium scan an imaging technique for identifying abscesses.

General anesthesia *see* Anesthesia, general.

General practitioner a physician who treats a wide variety of medical problems, usually referring patients to appropriate specialists where indicated.

Gland an aggregation of cells specialized to secrete or excrete materials not related to their ordinary metabolic needs; also called glandula.

Grading (prostatic carcinoma) the determination of a designator to index the degree of malignancy on the basis of microscopic appearance.

Hematuria blood in the urine.

> **Gross hematuria** urine in which blood is visible.

> **Microhematuria** urine in which blood is present but can only be seen by microscopic examination.

Hesitancy delayed initiation of the urinary stream.

Hormonal therapy reduction of the male hormone to castrate level to palliate prostate cancer.

Hormones those which are responsible for the secondary sex characteristics of men, predominantly testosterone.

Hyperplastic (prostatic) tissue *see* Benign prostatic hyperplasia.

Hypertrophy *see* Benign prostatic hypertrophy.

Hytrin (terazosin) a drug used in the treatment of hypertension that is helpful in relieving the symptoms of an enlarged prostate (BPH).

Immunoassay *see* Radioimmunoassay.

Impotence   the lack of ability of a male to initiate or maintain an erection of his penis that is sufficient for vaginal penetration.

Incontinence   the inability to control the voiding of urine.

> **Overflow**   the condition wherein the bladder retains urine after each voiding and therefore remains virtually full all or most of the time. The urine then involuntarily escapes from the full bladder by "spilling over."

> **Stress**   involuntary discharge of urine when there is an increase in the pressure within the bladder, as in coughing or straining.

> **Total**   failure of voluntary control of the sphincters (bladder neck and urethral) with constant or frequent involuntary passage of urine.

> **Urge**   the feeling of having to void that is so strong that it leads to an involuntary loss of urine (incontinence) if it is not relieved immediately.

Indium scans   *see* X-rays.

Indwelling catheterization   *see* Continuous, or indwelling, catheterization.

Infection   invasion by pathogenic microorganisms of a bodily part in which conditions are favorable for growth, production of toxins, and resulting injury to tissue.

Inflammation   redness, heat, swelling, or pain caused by irritation, injury, or infection.

Intermittency   stopping and starting of the urinary stream because of an inability to complete voiding and empty the bladder on one single contraction of the bladder.

Intermittent catheterization   catheterization, usually by one's self, on a systematic interval schedule in order to be certain that the bladder is emptied of *all* urine.

Internist   a physician whose specialty is internal medicine.

Isoenzymes   one of two or more chemically distinct but functionally identical forms of enzymes.

Lateral lobes (prostate)   *see* Lobes, prostate, lateral.

Lecithin granules   the granules found in prostatic secretions. They are decreased in bacterial infection in the prostate.

Lesion   a wound or injury.

> **Blastic**   increased density of bone seen on x-rays when there is extensive new bone formation due to cancerous destruction of bone.

Lytic decreased density of bone seen on x-rays when there has been destruction of bone by cancer.

Leydig cells the cells within the testis that produce testosterone.

Lithotomy position the position assumed by the patient in which he is flat on his back with the legs up in stirrups. This provides ready access to the perineum and genital area.

Lobes, prostate there are five distinct lobes of the prostate: two lateral, a middle, an anterior, and a posterior. Only the two lateral lobes and the middle lobe play a role in BPH.

Lateral the paired lobes of the prostate which often contribute to BPH.

Middle the commonest site of BPH, the middle lobe can never be felt on digital rectal examination.

Local anesthesia *see* Anesthesia, local.

Luteinizing hormone-releasing hormone (LH-RH) a hormone that initially acts on the testis to stimulate testosterone production, but then causes a cessation of testosterone production.

Lymph node a small mass of tissue in the form of an accumulation of lymphoid tissue. Lymph nodes serve as a defense mechanism for the body by removing bacteria and other toxins. They are also a common site of cancer spread.

Lytic lesion *see* Lesion, lytic.

Magnetic resonance imaging (MRI) similar to CT scanning in that cross-sectional images are obtained, an entirely new methodology for imaging. There is no ionizing radiation to which the patient is exposed and no known hazard to this imaging.

Male hormones the androgen hormones which are the masculinizing hormones, consisting of androsterone and testosterone.

Male reproductive system that part of the male concerned with the production, maturation, and transportation to the outside of the body of sperm.

Malignant tending to become progressively worse and to result in death; having the properties of invasion and metastases as applied to tumors.

Membrane a thin layer of tissue that covers a surface, lines a cavity, or divides a space.

Membranous urethra   *see* Urethra, membranous.

Mesoderm   one of the three primary derma layers of the embryo. The trigone of the bladder is derived from mesoderm.

Metastatic cancer   cancer that has spread outside the confines of the organ or structure in which it arose.

Metastasis   the spread of disease (cancer) from one organ or structure to another or to an area removed from the original site of the cancer.

Middle lobe (prostate)   *see* Lobes, prostate, middle.

Midstream (second-glass) urine   the urine from the middle of the voided stream with the initial and terminal parts of the stream voided elsewhere. The middle portion of the stream presumably contains urine from the bladder, the ureter, or the kidney but not from any portion of the urethra or bladder neck.

Nocturia   being awakened during the night by a desire to void.

Nonbacterial prostatitis   *see* Prostatitis, nonbacterial.

Nonspecific urethritis   *see* Urethritis, nonspecific.

Occult prostatic carcinoma   a carcinoma of the prostate that is neither suspected nor diagnosed but is discovered serendipitously after prostate surgery for BPH or after a biopsy triggered by an elevated PSA level. Also called stage A prostate cancer.

Orchiectomy   the surgical removal of a testis.
  Bilateral orchiectomy   the surgical removal of both testes.

Oval fat bodies   bodies found in prostatic secretions. They are increased in bacterial infection of the prostate.

Overflow incontinence   *see* Incontinence, overflow.

Peak urine flow rate   the maximum rate of flow, in milliliters per second, that a patient is able to generate.

Penile prosthesis   *see* Prosthesis, penile.

Penile (or pendulous) urethra   *see* Urethra, penile (or pendulous).

Perineal   pertaining to the perineum, the area of the body between the scrotum and the anus.

Posterior urethra   *see* Urethra, posterior.

Pressure/flow   a urodynamic test that is used to determine if a patient's symptoms are due to outlet obstruction or to a primary bladder problem.

Primary care physician   the first doctor to see an individual seeking medical care; the doctor also gives continuing medical care during health and illness. Examples are internists, pediatricians, family physicians, and obstetrician-gynecologists.

Primary sex gland   a gland necessary for reproduction. In the male, the testis is a primary gland.

Proscar (finasteride)   drug for the treatment of benign prostatic hyperplasia (BPH).

Prostate, or prostate gland   a gland in the male that surrounds the neck of the bladder and the first portion of the urethra as it leaves the bladder. Its principal function is to produce the majority of the fluid in which spermatozoa travel to the outside of the body. It also provides some of the nutrient material for the spermatozoa during their journey. The prostate is made up of connective tissue, muscle, and glandular tissue; it is the gland that manufactures the prostatic fluid.

Prostatic cancer   cancer arising in the prostate; it almost always arises within the glands that are in the prostate gland.

Prostate specific antigen (PSA)   a recently identified protein that is manufactured in the prostate gland. It is manufactured by both benign and malignant prostate cells.

Prostate surgery

Perineal   an approach to the prostate through the perineum; this approach is used for the treatment of BPH.

Radical perineal   an approach to the prostate through the perineum; this approach is used to treat prostate cancer. In this operation, the entire prostate gland is removed.

Radical retropubic   an approach through the lower abdomen and behind the pubic bone; this approach is used to treat prostate cancer. In this operation, the entire prostate gland is removed.

Retropubic   an approach through the lower abdomen and behind the pubic bone; this approach is used for the treatment of BPH. It is sometimes referred to as conservative retropubic prostatectomy.

Suprapubic   an approach through the lower abdomen and through the bladder; this approach is used to treat BPH.

Transurethral   a surgical approach through the urethra to relieve the symptoms of BPH.

Prostatic adenoma *see* Adenoma.

Prostatic biopsy *see* Biopsy.

Prostatic fossa *see* Fossa.

Prostatic massage (prostatic stripping) a digital rectal procedure whereby the index finger forcefully massages each of the two lateral lobes of the prostate for the purpose of obtaining secretions from the prostate gland. These secretions come out through the urethra.

Prostatic secretions *see* Secretions, prostatic.

Prostatic urethra *see* Urethra, prostatic.

Prostatitis

Bacterial, acute an inflammation of the prostate gland due to bacterial infection in which the patient is acutely ill.

Bacterial, chronic an inflammation of the prostate gland due to bacterial infection.

Nonbacterial inflammation in the prostate gland in the absence of any demonstrable bacterial organisms.

Prostatodynia pain in the perineal, rectal, or suprapubic area that is attributed to the prostate gland. In this condition the prostate gland is entirely normal.

Prostatostasis engorgement of the prostate gland with prostatic secretions due to irregular or infrequent orgasms and ejaculation. Also referred to as nonbacterial prostatitis.

Prosthesis (penile) a synthetic material that is inserted into the penis to make it rigid enough to allow for vaginal penetration. It is used for patients with erectile dysfunction (impotence).

Proteinuria the presence of protein in the urine. A small amount of protein in the urine (up to 200 milligrams per twenty-four hours) is normal; beyond that is considered abnormal.

Pubic symphysis the joint formed by a union of the pubic bones on the midline of the body by a thick mass of fibrous, cartilaginous material. It is the hard area felt by pressing firmly on the pubic hairline.

Pyuria the presence of white blood cells (pus cells) in the urine.

Radical prostatectomy the radical, or total, removal of the prostate gland that is done for the treatment of prostate cancer.

Radioimmunoassay an immunological technique for the measurement of minute quantities of antigen or antibodies, hormones, certain drugs, and other substances found within the body.

Radioisotope an isotope that is radioactive, thereby giving it the property of decay by one or more of several processes. Radioisotopes have important diagnostic and therapeutic uses in clinical medicine and research.

Rectal examination (prostate) the insertion of an examining finger into the rectum for the purpose of feeling the prostate gland.

Renal scans *see* Scans, renal.

Resection (transurethral) the removal of obstructing BPH prostate tissue that is done from within the urethra.

Resectoscope the instrument that is used for a transurethral resection.

Residual urine any urine that is left in the bladder immediately after voiding. The normal residual urine is 0 cubic centimeters.

Retention (urinary) the inability to void when the bladder is full. This is usually caused by obstruction to the flow of urine by the benign prostatic hyperplasia.

Retrograde ejaculation semen going backward into the bladder, instead of through the urethra to the outside, during orgasm and ejaculation. This is sometimes caused by an incomplete closure of the bladder neck during orgasm and ejaculation which frequently follows transurethral resection of the prostate gland.

Retropubic the area behind and below the pubic bone and pubic symphysis.

Scans (scanning)

Bone the production of a two-dimensional picture (a scan) representing the gamma rays emitted by a radioactive isotope concentrated in a specific tissue of the body, in this case the bone. When new bone is being laid down in a given area (a reparative phase) there is an increased uptake of the radioisotope in that area. The laying down of new bone may be in response to bone destruction from cancer spread to the bone, but it may also be in response to bone trauma or even to arthritis. An increased uptake of a radioisotope in one or more bones of a patient known to have prostatic cancer strongly suggests that the cancer has spread to those bones.

Renal the production of a two-dimensional picture (the scan) representing the gamma rays emitted by a radioactive isotope concentrated in a specific tissue of the body, in this case the kidney. Renal scans are used to determine blood flow to the kidney, kidney function, and obstruction to drainage of the kidney.

Scrotum the pouch, or sac, that contains the testes and their accessory organs.

Second-glass (midstream) urine the urine that is collected from the middle of the voided stream after the initial part of the urinary stream has been discarded and before the terminal part of the stream has been voided. Collection of only the middle portion of the urinary stream, or the second-glass urine, is a technique for examining the urine from the bladder, ureter, or kidney and for excluding possible bacterial contamination that might come from the urethra or the prostate.

Secretion, prostatic the fluid that is manufactured within the many glands of the prostate gland.

Semen the thick, whitish secretion of the reproductive organ in the male; it is composed of spermatozoa in their nutrient plasm, secretions from the prostate, seminal vesicles, and various other glands.

Seminal vesicle a pouch, or sac, that is a paired structure and located just behind the bladder. It provides nutrient material for the spermatozoa and may store spermatozoa as well. It empties into the prostatic urethra through the ejaculatory duct at the time of orgasm and ejaculation.

Seminiferous tubules the microscopic tubules within the testis where spermatozoa are manufactured.

Sexual dysfunction a less than normal functioning of the structure by which reproduction is achieved. An inability to achieve an erection, to maintain an erection, and to ejaculate are all examples of sexual dysfunction.

Sitz bath a small amount of water in the bottom of a bathtub that is just sufficient to cover the perineal area when a patient sits in it. When the water is warm and various bath salts are added to it, it can have a palliative effect on perineal pain or discomfort.

Spasm a sudden, violent, involuntary contraction of a muscle or a group of muscles.

Spermatozoa the mature male germ cell which is the specific output of the testes. It is the generative element of the semen, which serves to fertilize the ovum.

Sphincter (urinary) the muscle that can be voluntarily contracted to shut off the urinary system. In males it is located just beyond the prostate gland, going toward the penis, and the membranous portion of the urethra is enclosed within it.

Spinal anethesia *see* Anesthesia, spinal.

Spongy body lay term for the corpora cavernosa which are the structures within the penis that become engorged with blood during erection. When penile prostheses are used to treat individuals who are unable to achieve an erection, these paired prostheses are placed into the two corpora cavernosa of the penis so as to simulate the actual erectile process.

Staging (prostatic cancer) the process by which various tests are done to determine whether a prostatic cancer is still contained within the prostate gland or has spread outside of it.

Stress incontinence *see* Incontinence, stress.

Stricture, urethral a scarring or narrowing within the urethra that can produce symptoms of voiding difficulty very much like the symptoms of BPH. The stricture, or scar, within the urethra is often caused by an injury to a specific area within the urethra.

Suprapubic above, or superior to, the pubic symphysis and pubic bone. This term also refers to one of the surgical approaches for treatment of benign prostatic hyperplasia.

Surgical capsule (prostate) not a capsule at all but simply the interface between the benign prostatic hyperplasia and the true prostate gland. During surgery for the relief of BPH, all of the tissue inside this surgical capsule is removed; this leaves behind only the true prostate tissue.

Testosterone the principal circulating male hormone.

Third-glass urine (post–prostatic massage) the urine that is collected immediately following prostatic massage, which contains the secretions from the prostate gland that have pooled in the prostatic urethra. Examination of this third-glass urine is used to differentiate between infection in the urethra and infection in the prostate and between infection and simple inflammation within the prostate gland.

Tissue a collection of similar specialized cells united in the performance of a particular function.

Total incontinence *see* Incontinence, total.

Trabeculation (of the bladder) the condition of the bladder muscle when it has undergone a work buildup because of obstruction to the flow of urine from BPH. The buildup of the bladder muscle is irregular and induces a Swiss cheese appearance within the bladder consisting of very prominent bands of built-up muscle separated by recessed areas with no apparent buildup of the muscle. The appearance of trabeculation in the bladder is strong evidence of bladder outlet obstruction, usually due to benign prostatic hyperplasia.

Transurethral the route through the urethra. The term usually applies to something being passed into or through the urethra, as for example, a catheter, a cystoscope, or a resectoscope.

Trigone (bladder) *see* Bladder trigone.

True capsule (prostate) the fibrous layer of tissue that surrounds the true prostate tissue in much the same manner as the skin of an apple surrounds the pulp of the apple.

Tru-cut biopsy needle the traditional hollow lumen needle that is used to remove a "core," or "plug," of tissue from a solid structure, such as the prostate. The tissue is removed for microscopic examination to determine whether cancer is present.

True prostate tissue the substance of the normal prostate gland. It is made up of fibrous or connective tissue, muscle tissue, and glandular tissue.

Ultrasound (ultrasonography) a technique for the visualization of structures deep within the body by recording the echos of ultrasonic waves directed into the tissues. Ultrasonography is a noninvasive imaging technique for detecting masses within the body and for differentiating cystic masses from solid masses. It is also used as an aid in performing biopsies of the prostate.

Uremic poisoning (uremia) the retention and failure to eliminate excessive by-products of protein metabolism in the blood and the toxic condition produced thereby. It is characterized by nausea, vomiting, headache, dizziness, coma, or convulsions and, ultimately, death. The condition is usually caused by kidney failure.

Urethra the canal, or channel, through which urine is conveyed from the bladder to the exterior of the body. It is divided into anatomic areas beginning at the bladder neck.
  Bulbous the portion of the urethra that begins at the end of the membranous urethra and continues to the penile, or

pendulous, portion of the urethra. It has the largest diameter of any portion of the urethra.

Membranous the portion of the urethra contained within the external urethral sphincter. It begins at the end of the prostatic urethra and ends at the beginning of the bulbous urethra.

Penile (or pendulous) the portion of the urethra contained within the penis.

Posterior the prostatic urethra and the membranous urethra taken together.

Prostatic the portion of the urethra beginning at the bladder neck and ending at the external urethral sphincter. It is contained entirely within the prostate gland.

Urethral stricture *see* Stricture, urethral.

Urethritis, nonspecific infection in the posterior urethra that can be caused by any microorganism except gonococcus.

Urge incontinence *see* Incontinence, urge.

Urgency the strong feeling of having to void that, if not relieved promptly, will lead to incontinence.

Urinary sphincter *see* Sphincter, urinary.

Urine analysis the physical, chemical, and microscopic analysis and examination of urine.

Urine culture the incubation of urine at a specific temperature and in a specific medium so as to permit the growth and identification of microorganisms. This is the definitive means by which an infection in the urinary tract is diagnosed.

Urodynamic studies quantitative means by which the two principal functions of the bladder, consisting of urine storage and urine evacuation, can be measured.

Urologist a physician who specializes in the medical and surgical treatment of diseases of the urinary tract in males and females and the reproductive tract in males. A urologist must have had at least five years of hospital training following graduation from medical school and passed the written and oral examinations given by the American Board of Urology.

Urothelium the lining of any portion of the urinary tract.

Vas deferens the muscular, tubular structure that propels and transports spermatozoa from the epididymis into the prostatic urethra.

Weak urinary stream   a voided stream that has less than normal expulsive force to it. This can be quantified by measuring the maximum urinary flow rate expressed in milliliters per second.

Work hypertrophy (of the bladder)   the muscle buildup that occurs within the bladder in response to the new growth of BPH tissue which makes bladder emptying more difficult. The actual buildup of muscle within the bladder is called trabeculation.

X-rays   electromagnetic vibrations of short wavelengths that can penetrate most substances to some extent and reveal the presence and position of fractures or foreign bodies. They can also cause some substances to fluoresce, by which the size, shape, and movement of various organs can be observed.

INDEX

10-30
150